W9-CDC-444

Medical Imaging Systems Techniques and Applications

Cardiovascular Systems

Gordon and Breach International Series in Engineering, Technology and Applied Science

Edited by Cornelius T. Leondes

Books on **Medical Imaging Systems Techniques and Applications**

Forthcoming in the *Gordon and Breach International Series in Engineering, Technology and Applied Science*

Structural Dynamic Systems Computational Techniques and Optimization

Mechatronics Systems Techniques and Applications

Biomechanic Systems Techniques and Applications

Computer Aided and Integrated Manufacturing Systems Techniques and Applications

Expert Systems Techniques and Applications

This book is part of a series. The publisher will accept continuation orders which may be cancelled at any time and which provide for automatic billing and shipping of each title in the series upon publication. Please write for details.

Medical Imaging Systems Techniques and Applications

Cardiovascular Systems

Edited by

Cornelius T. Leondes

Professor Emeritus
University of California
at Los Angeles

Gordon and Breach Science Publishers

Australia • Canada • China • France • Germany • India • Japan •
Luxembourg • Malaysia • The Netherlands • Russia • Singapore •
Switzerland • Thailand • United Kingdom

Amsteldijk 166
1st Floor
1079 LH Amsterdam
The Netherlands

British Library Cataloguing in Publication Data

Medical imaging systems techniques and applications
    Cardiovascular systems. — (Gordon and Breach international
    series in engineering, technology and applied science ; v.
    1)
    1. Cardiovascular system — Imaging
    I. Leondes, Cornelius T.
    616.1'0754

ISBN 90-5699-509-X

CONTENTS

SERIES DESCRIPTION AND MOTIVATION

Many aspects of explosively growing technology are difficult or essentially impossible for one author to treat in an adequately comprehensive manner. Spectacular technological growth is made stunningly manifest by any number of examples, but, just to note one here, the Intel 486 IBM-compatible PC was first introduced in late 1989. At that time the price of this PC was in the $10,000 range and it was thought to be much too powerful for widespread use. By early 1992, a little more than two years later, the price had dropped to $1,000 and it was felt that much more power was needed, leading directly to the Pentium IBM-compatible PC. A similar price reduction pattern has already been projected for the Pentium computer, and, in view of the recent history of the 486, it is difficult to suggest that the same "power hungry" pattern will not occur again in a similar time span. In any event, this example and its clear implications with respect to the many application-oriented issues in diverse fields of engineering, technology, and applied science and their continuing advances make it obvious that this series will fill an essential role in numerous ways for individuals and organizations.

Areas of major significance will be defined and world-class co-authors identified as contributors for essential volumes in respective areas. These areas will be determined by criteria including:

1. Will volumes fill important textbook voids in respective areas?
2. In some cases, a "time void" for an important area will clearly suggest the need for a volume. For example, the important area of Expert Systems might have a textbook void of several years that "requires" an important new volume.
3. Are these technology areas that simply cannot sensibly be treated comprehensively by a single author or even several co-authors?

Examples of areas requiring important volumes will be carefully defined and structured and might include, as the case arises, volumes in:

1. Medical imaging
2. Mechatronics
3. Computer network techniques and applications

4. Multimedia techniques and applications
5. CAD/CAE (Computer Aided Design/Computer Aided Engineering)
6. FEA (Finite Element Analysis) techniques and applications
7. Computational techniques in structural dynamic systems
8. Neural networks (as might possibly be suggested by a significant time void in the textbook literature)
9. Expert Systems (again, depending on a possible significant time void).

One of the most important aspects of this series will be that, despite rapid advances in technology, respective volumes will be defined and structured to constitute works of indefinite or "lasting" reference interest.

SERIES PREFACE

The first industrial revolution, with its roots in James Watt's steam engine and its various applications to modes of transportation, manufacturing and other areas, introduced to mankind novel ways of working and living, thus becoming one of the chief determinants of our present way of life.

The second industrial revolution, with its roots in modern computer technology and integrated electronics technology — particularly VLSI (Very Large Scale Integrated) electronics technology, has also resulted in advances of enormous significance in all areas of modern activity, with great economic impact as well.

Some of the areas of modern activity created by this revolution are: medical imaging, structural dynamic systems, mechatronics, biomechanics, computer-aided and integrated manufacturing systems, applications of expert and knowledge-based systems, and so on. Documentation of these areas well exceeds the capabilities of any one or even several individuals, and it is quite evident that single-volume treatments — whose intent would be to provide practitioners with useful reference sources — while useful, would generally be rather limited.

It is the intent of this series to provide comprehensive multi-volume treatments of areas of significant importance, both the above-mentioned and others. In all cases, contributors to these volumes will be individuals who have made notable contributions in their respective fields. Every attempt will be made to make each book self-contained, thus enhancing its usefulness to practitioners in a specific area or related areas. Each multi-volume treatment will constitute a well-integrated but distinctly titled set of volumes. In summary, it is the goal of the respective sets of volumes in this series to provide an essential service to the many individuals on the international scene who are deeply involved in contributing to significant advances in the second industrial revolution.

PREFACE

Medical Imaging Systems Techniques and Applications

Because of the availability of powerful computational techniques, new modality techniques such as Computer-Aided Tomography (CAT), Magnetic Resonance Imaging (MRI) and others, and because of the new techniques of imaging processing (machine vision), the lives of many patients will be saved, and the quality of all our lives improved. This marriage of powerful computer technology and medical imaging has spawned a new and growing generation of young dynamic doctors who hold PhDs in physics and/or computer science, along with their MDs. In addition, technologists and computer scientists, with their superb skills, are also deeply involved contributors to this area of major significance. Thus, medical imaging systems is a most appropriate and very diversely broad subject area of major international importance with which to initiate this *Gordon and Breach International Series in Engineering, Technology and Applied Science*. This subject area exemplifies a meaningful manifestation of the power of the technologies of the second industrial revolution. Further, it illustrates interdisciplinary trends — including career development — that are an inevitable by-product of such technologies.

The first set of volumes on *Medical Imaging Systems Techniques and Applications* consists of 6 distinctly titled and well-integrated volumes, that can nevertheless be utilized as individual books. Needless to say, however, the great breadth of this field certainly suggests the requirement for at least 6 volumes for a relatively comprehensive treatment. It might also be remarked at this time that because of the rapidly expanding advances in this broad discipline, it will, in all likelihood, be appropriate to address this field again several years from now with another set of reference volumes.

In any event, the set of volumes on medical imaging treats:

1. Cardiovascular Systems
2. Brain and Skeletal Systems
3. Diagnosis Optimization Techniques
4. General Anatomy
5. Modalities
6. Computational Techniques.

The first chapter in this volume on cardiovascular systems emphasizes the importance of accurate measurements of cardiac shape and dynamics as they reflect the scope of cardiac diseases, the major cause of mortality in developed countries today. Cardiac imaging plays an important role in this regard, and almost the only one in this clinical context. Azhari, Beyar and Sideman present an in-depth treatment of the issues involved in this field, with many important areas covered. Just to mention one, most past studies have been based on two-dimensional (2-D) data sets that discard the true three-dimensional (3-D) cardiac geometry and obviously result in considerable error. But many other issues are covered in this chapter and, as a result, it is a most appropriate beginning to the volume.

Abd-El-Ouahab Boudraa provides a thorough review of the techniques used to assess the Left Ventricle Function (LVF) in chapter 2. The various modalities utilized for this vital function are considered and compared. Further, this chapter contains an extensive compilation of the literature in this field. As a result, it will undoubtedly constitute a unique reference in this major area.

The problem of image sequence filtering in clinical angiography with quantum limited scenes is addressed by Cheuk L. Chan, A. K. Katsaggelos and A. V. Sahakian (chapter 3). It is essential to develop quality images for effective diagnosis or analysis, while at the same time lowering x-ray dosages traditionally utilized in practice. New highly effective techniques in filtering and displacement field estimation in quantum mottle are presented here. Other issues and techniques are dealt with in this treatment of techniques in clinical angiography. A comprehensive bibliography is included.

Chapter 4 by Milan Sonka and Steve M. Collins informs us that at present, every year about 1.5 million people with coronary artery disease, in the United States alone, suffer from myocardial infarction. The death rate from coronary artery disease itself is currently in excess of 500,000 per year. Coronary angiography has maintained a pivotal role in the evaluation and treatment of patients with coronary disease; hundreds of thousands of coronary angiograms are performed annually, in just the United States. The vast majority of these angiograms are interpreted visually; this does not necessarily allow for the requisite accuracy in the assessment of the physiological significance of coronary obstructions. This chapter covers issues concerning and techniques to be used for the more effective treatment of this international problem. Particular attention is given to reliable automated analysis of coronary angiograms. A substantial bibliography is included.

The final chapter in this book reviews intravascular ultrasound imaging techniques for evaluating coronary artery anatomy. Because of its special and effective techniques it is entirely possible, if not probable, that intravascular ultrasound imaging may ultimately replace angiography as the "gold standard" in evaluating coronary artery disease. And because of the great impact of this field on the international scene, this chapter by Sonka, McKay and von Birgelen is a most appropriate conclusion to this unique volume.

This book on cardiovascular systems imaging techniques clearly reveals the effectiveness and significance of the techniques available and, with further development, the essential role they will play in the future. The authors are all to be highly commended for their splendid contributions; these papers will serve as an important and unique reference for students, research workers, practitioners, computer scientists and many others on the international scene for years to come.

1 THREE DIMENSIONAL ANALYSIS OF HEART GEOMETRY AND FUNCTION

HAIM AZHARI,* RAFAEL BEYAR and SAMUEL SIDEMAN

*Heart System Research Center, The Julius Silver Institute,
Department of Biomedical Engineering,
Technion-Israel Institute of Technology,
Haifa, 32000, Israel*

1.1. INTRODUCTION

The heart is an organ that functions by a periodic change of its three dimensional (3D) shape. The pumping function of the heart is characterized by a highly temporally ordered periodic change of the 3D spatial geometry of the heart's chambers. The instantaneous cardiac shape is an important parameter which reflects on the complex shape-function interactions of the electric, metabolic, neural and mechanical control systems. It determines the blood volume enclosed within its main cavities, namely the left ventricle (LV) and the right ventricle (RV), and couples between the blood pressure and the myocardial strains (e.g., through the Law of Laplace[1]).

The LV shape changes determine the blood flow to the aorta and consequently the LV blood pressure and the coronary flow. The most evident manifestations of the shape-function relationship may be observed in developed cardiac pathologies[2-8] such as fibrous aneurysms, ischemic scars and others; these are usually manifested by the global changes of cardiac shape (e.g., dilatation of the ventricles, thin aneurysmal walls) as well as by abnormal cardiac motion.[2,3,5] While these can be based

---

*Correspondence: Haim Azhari, D.Sc., Dept. of Biomedical Engineering, Technion-IIT, Haifa 32000, Israel. Fax: 972 4 8234131.

on comparing LV wall thickness and motion only between end-diastole (ED) and end-systole (ES), the temporal sequence of contraction may highlight cardiac pathologies.[9,10] Thus, by quantitatively analyzing the heart's geometry and its temporal changes one can characterize the functional state of the heart and learn to distinguish between normal and abnormal conditions.[11]

In vivo heart geometry is best defined by imaging. However, in most previous studies are based on two dimensional (2D) data sets and therefore discard the true 3D cardiac geometry which obviously results in considerable errors.[9,12–14] In this chapter we review and assess some available 3D imaging methodologies for the quantitative analysis and assessment of the normal and pathological heart shape-function relationship.

1.2. CARDIAC IMAGING METHODS

1.2.1. Imaging and Visualization

Imaging denotes the art of converting normally unseen phenomena into observable, visual, entities. Unlike *visualization*, which identifies normally unseen objects by tracers or otherwise, *imaging* involves reconstructing the physical entity from data sets generated by the imaging technique. As imaging involves visualization, these two terms are commonly interchanged. Here we consider "imaging" in the broad all inclusive sense of this term.

The outstanding progress in computer technology and image processing techniques allows us to address, simulate and analyze the shape-function relationships in the complicated spatio-temporal 3D systems. Of particular importance is the interplay between the visual entity which provides a quantitative understanding of the studied phenomena, and the quantitative information contained within the visual images. The dynamic field, which represents a spatio-temporal behavior of some parameter, can either be mapped directly by the imaging system as with infrared image sequences, or estimated and reconstructed from appropriate measurement data. The latter is the case of the dynamic 3D cardiac wall thickness which is based on edge detection algorithms and geometrical data. Thus, a data processing stage must precede the visualization stage in most cases, with vectorial data providing topological information from critical field points and connecting surfaces and tensorial data providing streamlines and isosurfaces.

This review relates to unravelling of the cardiac shape-function relationships, which are based on three dimensional (3D) imaging techniques. A short review of the presently available imaging modalities will help put this objective in proper perspective.

1.2.2. Imaging Modalities

The oldest procedure of cardiac imaging is, of course, thoracic X-ray, in which the heart is projected as a dark shadow within the rib cage. The interpretation of the image is mainly qualitative in nature. As the attenuation of X-rays by soft tissue is rather low, the contrast is poor and the obtained images indicate only whether the heart is "normal", or deviates abnormally from the typical normal size.

Contrast agents improve image resolution. Angiography, first reported by Forssman,[15] combines catheterization with injection of contrast agents to the heart cavities or coronary vessels, and provides clear images of the coronary tree and fair images of the heart's cavities. Angiography, the leading method for detecting coronary artery diseases, is an invasive procedure and involves some risk to the patient. Exposure to non-negligible doses of X-ray radiation during angiography may have a small but definite consequence.

Cardiac ultrasonic imaging, i.e., *echocardiography*, is completely noninvasive and can therefore be used frequently. Moreover, echocardiography can yield dynamic images of cross-sections of the heart and, combined with color Doppler, provides overlay maps of blood flow patterns. These features make echocardiography the most commonly used imaging modality. However, echocardiography has three major disadvantages: (i) imaging is limited to certain viewing windows (i.e., the intercostal spaces) (ii) image quality is typically fair and (iii) image resolution decreases with range and is in the order of 2–3 mm. While transesophageal echocardiography[16] overcomes the first limitation, the other two limitations remain.

An exciting and clinically promising ultrasonic technology involves intravascular echography.[17] Though invasive in nature, this procedure allows to view the stenotic regions in the coronaries and thus greatly affects the therapeutic procedure.

Radioactive based imaging techniques such as the Gamma-Camera, single photon emission tomography (SPECT) and positron emission tomography (PET) permit the *in vivo* application of tracer kinetic principles. Tracer amounts of isotope-labelled compounds are administered intravenously or by inhalation, allowing to derive clinically significant temporal or spatial information on the tracer concentration and activity in the tissue. Tracer kinetic models can relate the temporal changes in the tracers' concentration to metabolic rates, regional myocardial blood flow and oxygen consumption. High temporal resolution of modern PET scanners allows to quantify the relationship between substrate delivery, transmembrane transport and intracellular substrate utilization, and the spatial distribution and heterogeneity of these processes in the normal and diseased myocardium can be mapped and evaluated.[18] Unfortunately, the relatively poor spatial resolution of these techniques prohibits relating these functions to the true geometry of the heart. Other sophisticated imaging tools such as computer tomography (CT) and magnetic resonance (MR) are therefore needed when searching for the shape-function relationships in the cardiac muscle.

The introduction of fast CT techniques into cardiology involved shortening the data acquisition time to several milliseconds, and obtaining sequential exposures representing one heart beat. Two techniques are presently available: the digital spatial reconstructor (DSR)[19] and the Cine-CT.[20] Both techniques provide high spatial resolution images (pixels of about 1 mm in size) with high quality and high temporal resolution. However, these techniques expose the patient to relatively high doses of X-ray radiation and require intravenous injection of contrast material. Furthermore, these techniques typically provide only sets of short axis images taken by "slicing" the long axis of the heart.

Magnetic resonance imaging (MRI), is noninvasive and the magnetic field involved in the measurement does not cause any detrimental effects on the tissue. It can provide images along any arbitrarily selected plane and may provide high quality, high resolution data. Sufficient temporal resolution is obtained either by applying ECG gated acquisition or by using rapid acquisition methods (e.g., echo-planar,[21] or spiral imaging[22]). In addition, MRI can be applied in 3D imaging on the entire volume contouring the heart. It can be used along with contrast materials to depict perfusion maps, and along with MR spectroscopy to provide metabolic information. Moreover, MRI has a unique feature: the ability to noninvasively tag certain regions of the myocardium.[23,24] Finally, recent developments in the field involve MR coronary angiography, which may become a revolution in diagnostic catheterization once resolution and motion problems are overcome. MRI is a most effective and versatile imaging tool available today, but high operation costs are still a major factor hindering its wide clinical application in cardiology.

1.3. DATA MANAGEMENT

One can roughly divide the imaging data sets into four major categories:

(i) Projection type images: Information is obtained from shadows of semi-transparent objects; this is typical of X-ray angiography and some radioactive based imaging techniques.

(ii) Multi-slice parallel plane images: This is typical of the tomographic techniques (Figure 1A).

(iii) Axially rotated images: Images are typically obtained along planes rotated around the LV long axis, as in apical echocardiography[25] (Figure 1B).

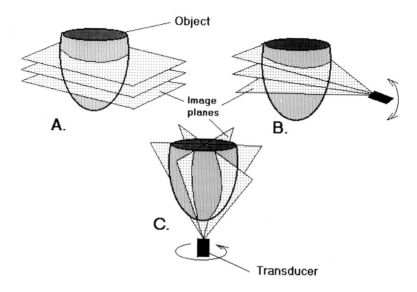

Figure 1. Typical imaging data sets available for 3D computer reconstruction of the heart. (A) Multi-slice parallel plane images. (B) Axially rotated images. (C) Arbitrarily oriented planes.

(iv) Arbitrarily oriented planes: Cross-sectional images of the heart are obtained along arbitrarily oriented planes. This category is typical of 2D echocardiography, and can also be implemented in MRI, though less frequently than category (ii). Note that in 3D echocardiography the spatial orientation of each plane is known either by using a spark system[26] or by applying an iterative matching procedure[27] (Figure 1C).

Another classification of data management relates to stationary (or rather quasistationary) data and dynamic data. The quasistationary data is usually taken at well defined reproducible temporal or spatial end-points in the cardiac cycle. The most common points of reference are the end-diastolic (ED) and end-systolic (ES) states, which are commonly used as reference points to study changes during the entire cardiac cycle and for comparison between different hearts. The dynamic data is taken either continuously, as in the case of tracers, or intermittently during the cycle, thus presenting a finite sequence of images between ES and ED.

Practically all the work reported here relates to the analysis of the stationary and the intermittent-dynamic cardiac data.

1.4. TWO DIMENSIONAL (2D) LEFT VENTRICULAR SHAPE ANALYSES

The first quantitative analysis of the LV geometry is probably due to Woods[28] who in 1892 applied the Laplace equation to incised and preserved hearts. In its simplest form the Laplace equation states that:

$$\sigma = P \cdot \frac{R}{2T} \tag{1}$$

where σ is the stress induced in the myocardial wall, P is the LV cavity blood pressure, T is the wall thickness and R is the LV radius of curvature. As can be concluded from Equation (1), the geometrical factor R/T determines the stress within the myocardium which "resists" contraction. This equation can provide a general explanation why dilated hearts are weaker, as a larger R induces a larger σ and why pathological high pressure results in hypertrophy of the wall, i.e., σ decreases as T increases.

Woods' quantitative approach gained clinical acceptance[29,30] and the curvature/thickness ratio, R/T, was investigated *in vitro*[31] and *in vivo*[32] using angiographic or echocardiographic images, and recently, 3D MRI.

Quantitative assessment of the LV by assuming spherical or ellipsoidal geometries is convenient but insufficient, as the LV radius of curvature varies with location. Gibson and Brown[33] suggested a non-dimensional 2D shape index (SI), which can be used to quantify the roundness of the LV shape.

$$SI = \frac{4\pi A}{p^2} \tag{2}$$

where p is the LV shape perimeter and A is its area. SI equals unity for a perfect circular shape and has values <1 for elliptic shapes. The advantage here is that this index relates to the entire LV shape and does not rely on regional measurements. However, this index is not directional, and longitudinal and lateral elongation of the LV can yield identical SI value.

A more directional "eccentricity" index (E), was suggested by Fischel *et al.*:[34]

$$E = \frac{(L^2 - D^2)^{1/2}}{L} \tag{3}$$

where L is the LV major axis and D is the LV minor axis, both measured from angiographic projection images. Obviously, $E = 0$ for a perfect sphere and its value increases as the heart becomes more elongated ($E = 1$ for a straight vertical line).

Azancot et al.[35] suggested the application of the Fourier transform to the traced echocardiographic 2D cross-section images of the LV. This approach was adopted by Kass et al.,[36] who implemented spectral indices to angiographically obtained contours. They have shown that the shape characteristics of LVs with aortic regurgitation differ significantly from that of normal hearts. A slightly different approach was suggested by Duvernoy et al.[37] who have replaced the Fourier transform representation by a Fourier descriptor for closed curves. Their descriptor has the advantage of being insensitive to translation, rotation and scaling of the image.

Marcus et al.[38] compared a number of quantitative methods for characterizing LV contraction based on 2D angiographic data and proposed a rather unique curvature dependent approach to the shape analysis. Halmann et al.[10] extended this procedure and proposed a dynamic analysis of the LV shape based on the curvature function.

1.5. THREE DIMENSIONAL (3D) SHAPE ANALYSIS

1.5.1. Shape Characterization

The obvious disadvantage of all 2D procedures for characterizing the LV shape is that they discount the 3D geometry of the heart and thus yield erroneous results. However, early attempts to characterize the heart's 3D geometry have either used geometrical assumptions about the shape to reach conclusions about the shape,[39] or were too cumbersome for practical use (e.g., the multi-chart approach by Janicki et al.,[40] or the spherical harmonics by Schundy et al.[41]). With the advancement of new imaging modalities such as Cine-CT and MRI, in vivo data covering the entire heart can be obtained and utilized to investigate the in situ 3D geometry. Typical Cine-CT scans are depicted in Figure 2.

1.5.2. The Geometrical-Cardiogram (GCG)

A novel procedure for describing the spatial geometry of the LV by using a special helical shape descriptor was suggested by Azhari et al.[42,43] The procedure assumes that the LV is enclosed within an imaginary cylinder with a diameter larger than the larger diameter of the LV. Moving along a helical path on the cylinder (Figure 3), and measuring the radial distance R from the surface of the cylinder to the endocardial (or epicardial) surface of the LV, yields a function $R(\xi)$ which describes a spatial curve wrapped around the LV shape and can be used to approximate its geometry. It is important to note that the accuracy of this 3D description is inversely proportional to the helical step H_0 and the description is exact when $H_0 \rightarrow 0$.

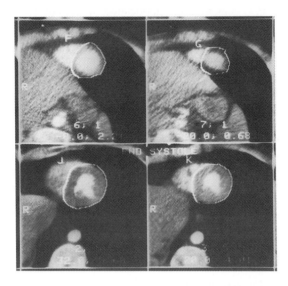

Figure 2. Four typical Cine-CT cross-section images of a human heart. Ten to twelve such cross-sections are commonly required to cover the entire heart with an interslice distance of about 1 cm. Note that the LV epicardial boundary is traced in these images.

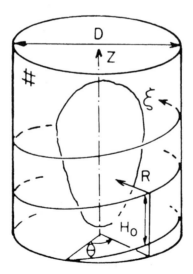

Figure 3. Schematics of the enclosing cylinder and coordinate system utilized to obtain the helical shape descriptor (printed with permission from Azhari et al.[42] ©1987 IEEE).

The major advantage of the derived function $R(\xi)$ is that it describes the 3D geometry by a unidimensional vector, and common unidimensional signal processing operators (e.g., filters and transformations) can be readily applied to manipulate the spatial geometry.

Keeping the number of windings needed to reach the base from the apex constant assures that each point along the helix retains its relative height, regardless of the size of the heart. Furthermore, the LV long axis is aligned with the imaginary cylinder axis, and the direction connecting the long axis and the middle of the septal wall is defined as the reference direction from which the helix begins. Thus, each point along $R(\xi)$ retains its relative circumferential position regardless of the size of the heart. Finally the length of the path along $R(\xi)$ is normalized, so it is zero at the apex and 1 at the base and the lateral dimensions are normalized by the length of the LV long axis. (The normalized helical coordinate is denoted as η and the normalized radial coordinate is denoted as ρ.) The ensuing nondimensional helical vector $\rho(\eta)$ which describes the normalized 3D geometry of the LV, is denoted "geometrical cardiogram" (GCG).[43,44]

The ability of the GCG to describe the geometrical features of the studied 3D object regardless of the object's size, is easily demonstrated by applying the GCG to sets of well defined geometries (cylinders, spheres, ellipsoids). Indeed, all the cylinders yield an identical GCG which looks like a step function; the cones yield an identical ramp-like GCG signal, and all spheres and all ellipsoids with the same aspect ratio yield typical GCG signals, regardless of their size.

A set of GCG signals obtained for a group of normal human hearts at ED is depicted in Figure 4. The similarity between these "normal" signals under normal conditions suggests that the features of the normal GCG pattern can be characterized quantitatively and, consequently, that GCG signals from abnormal hearts which have a distorted geometry could be identified as significantly different from the normal pattern. This distinction is achieved by utilizing a "shape distortion index" (SDI) which is based on the Karhunen-Loeve Transform (KLT).[44]

Given a set of N dimensional characteristic pattern vectors $\{\bar{\rho}\}$ which represent the GCG signals typical to the normal population, it is possible to expand every vector $\bar{\rho}$ from the set by an arbitrary yet complete set of orthonormal basis vectors $\bar{\Phi}$, without loosing any information. However, when only the first K basis functions of the expansion are used, an approximation $\hat{\rho}$ of the expanded vector $\bar{\rho}$ is obtained:

$$\hat{\rho} = \sum_{j=1}^{K} C_j \bar{\Phi}_j + \bar{M}_\rho \tag{4}$$

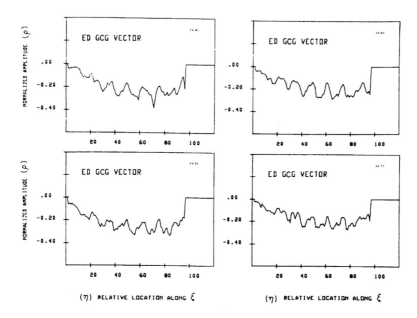

Figure 4. A typical set of GCG signals obtained for four different normal human LV's at ED (printed with permission from Azhari et al.[44] © 1989 IEEE).

where C_j designates the coefficient associated with the basis vector $\bar{\Phi}_j$, and $M_j = E\{\bar{\rho}\}$ is the mean vector of the set; ($E\{\bar{\rho}\}$ is the expected value operator). The discrepancy between the original vector $\bar{\rho}$ and its approximation $\hat{\rho}$ is evaluated by the mean square error (MSE), which is given by:

$$\text{MSE} = E\{\|\bar{\rho} - \hat{\rho}\|^2\} \tag{5}$$

The most unique feature of the KLT is that for any number of K terms used in Equation (4), the approximated vector $\hat{\rho}$ has the minimal possible MSE. The KLT is optimal in the sense that it compresses the information into uncorrelated basis vectors with a descending degree of importance. Unlike the Fourier and other transforms, the basis vectors $\bar{\Phi}_j$ are not known *a priori* but are "tailor made" for the studied reference population.

1.5.3. The Shape Distortion Index

The KLT can be utilized to discriminate between normal and pathological hearts based on their 3D geometry.[44] This involves obtaining a set of KLT

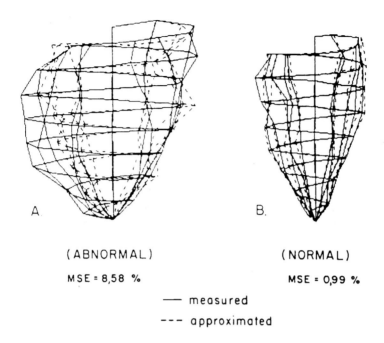

A   B.

(ABNORMAL)   (NORMAL)

MSE = 8,58 %   MSE = 0,99 %

—— measured

--- approximated

Figure 5. 3D wireframe reconstructions of two human LVs demonstrating the implication of different MSE values. The solid line corresponds to the measured data and the dashed line to its corresponding KLT approximation. (A) Abnormal LV (B) Normal LV. Note the large discrepancy between the measured and approximated shapes in the abnormal case with contrast to the close approximation obtained for the normal LV (printed with permission from Azhari et al.[44] © 1989 IEEE).

basis functions for the endocardial ED and ES of the reference normal group and for a group of patients with a cardiac disease. The MSE for the abnormal hearts are consistently larger than the MSE for normal hearts. A typical 3D reconstruction of a normal LV and an abnormal one are compared to their KLT reconstructions in Figure 5. Note the much larger discrepancy for the abnormal heart. Optimization yields that the first four ES KLT basis functions have the best discriminatory power.[44] The distortion of the pathological heart in comparison to the normal one can be quantified by defining the shape distortion index (SDI):

$$SDI = \frac{MSE_p - \mu_n}{\sigma_n} \tag{6}$$

where MSE is based on the first four ES KLT basis functions for the particular heart under study, μ_n and σ_n are, respectively, the average and MSE values obtained for the group of normal hearts. Note that by definition the expected SDI value for normal hearts is zero, and assuming a Gaussian distribution for the SDI values, a heart with an SDI > 3 may be categorically considered abnormal ($p < 0.04$). The SDI values for the group of abnormal hearts ranged between 8.61 to 17.32,[44] indicating that the suggested technique has clinical merit.

The KLT based shape distortion analysis is also useful in localizing regional abnormalities,[45] as in hearts with aneurysm. The regional shape deviation from the expected normal shape is determined by evaluating the KLT reconstruction error for each point along the GCG vector. Thus, the GCG obtained by the KLT based shape analysis may not only detect hearts with aneurysm but also locate the aneurysmal regions.

1.5.4. Sorting Pathological Hearts

The ability to distinguish between normal and ischemic hearts by the GCG based shape analysis[12] led to investigate the possibility of using the GCG to sort between abnormal hearts with different pathologies.[46] As is well known, different geometric distortions may be generated by different pathologies. However, the GCG spectral decomposition may help in sorting the different diseases by determining their geometrical characteristics.

As shown by Azhari et al.,[46] the GCG can be expressed analytically by a Fourier-sine series:

$$\text{GCG} = \tilde{\rho}(\eta) = \sum_{n=1}^{\infty} A_n \cdot \sin(n\pi\eta) \quad 0 \leq \eta \leq 1 \tag{7}$$

where A_n designates the amplitude of the nth harmonic, and $\eta = 0$ corresponds to the apex and $\eta = 1$ to the LV base. Since the left hand side of Equation (7) represents a 3D shape, each harmonic on the right hand side must also represent a 3D shape.

Consider the first harmonic. If A_1 is not zero, then moving along η from apex to base describes a helical trajectory in space which encloses a football shape (Figure 6A). Mathematically this shape is obtained by rotating a single lobe of a sine function with amplitude A_1 around the LV long axis. As the absolute value of A_1 is increased, the shape grows in the lateral direction. Decreasing A_1 yields a laterally narrower shape, assuming the form of a cigar. Note that due to the definitions of the GCG, an harmonic with $A_1 < 0$ describes a real object, and an harmonic with $A_1 > 0$ describes a "hole" in space with a shape similar to the one described.

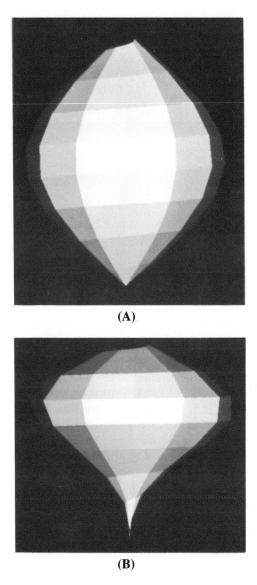

(A)

(B)

Figure 6. The 3D interpretation of the GCG spectral decomposition. (A) 3D reconstruction of the GCG first harmonic. Note that for $A_1 < 0$, this shape corresponds to a real object while, for $A_1 > 0$, this shape corresponds to a "hole" in space. (B) 3D reconstruction of the GCG first and second harmonics. (C) 3D reconstruction of the GCG first and third harmonics. Note that a different shape is obtained if A_3 and A_1 differ in signs.

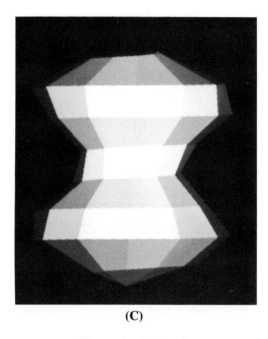

(C)

Figure 6. *Continued.*

Next, consider the second harmonic. The shape described by this harmonic has two lobes, like two footballs spiked on the LV long axis. As the two lobes differ in the signs of their amplitude, one describes a real object while the other describes a "hole" in space. To depict this geometry we combine it with a real object defined by the first harmonic. The result is a "tear-drop" shape (Figure 6B), which points upward or downward, depending on the sign of A_2; in normal hearts the "tear-drop" points upward.

Finally, consider the third harmonic. This harmonic has three lobes, "spiked" along the LV long axis, representing a real part at the top and a real part at the bottom and a "hole" in the center, or vice versa. The results of combining the third and first harmonics are depicted in Figure 6C for the case common to normal human hearts.

The spectral decomposition of the GCG allows to determine the geometrical regularity of the shape. As shown,[46] the contribution of each harmonic to the volume enclosed by the LV shape is proportional to the square of its amplitude; higher harmonics correspond to the more complicated features of the studied shape. Consequently, the higher the relative contribution of the lower harmonics to the volume of the studied shape, the more regular it is. The geometrical regularity index (GR_M) allows to quantify this feature:

$$GR_M = \frac{\sum_{n=1}^{M} A_n^2}{\sum_{n=1}^{\infty} A_n^2} \qquad (8)$$

where M is the number of lower harmonics used. Note that GR_M equals 1 if the shape is exactly defined by the first M harmonics. GR_M is smaller for less regular shapes.

Using the amplitudes of the first three harmonics, i.e., A_1, A_2, A_3, and the geometrical regularity index GR_M for $M = 8$ in Equation (8), suffices to characterize human hearts. The results are depicted in the A_1–A_3–GR_8 parametric space for 10 normal hearts, nine aneurysmal hearts, five with myocardial infarction and three with hypertrophy, in Figure 7. As seen, each pathology has its own cluster. Automatic classification of these hearts was obtained by an algorithm for unsupervised clustering,[46] with an overall success of 85%, suggesting that GCG based shape analysis is sensitive enough to allow for computerized clinical applications. Note that the discrimination between hearts with aneurysm and myocardial infarctions is rather vague, since aneurysm evolves from myocardial infarction resulting with a continuous cluster of the two groups in Figure 7.

1.5.5. MRI Tagging

The use of the helical coordinate system, which can account for long axis shortening, allows to map ischemic regions on the myocardium. However, the heart contracts longitudinally as well as radially, and twists substantially. Thus, to fully describe this 3D complicated phenomena one must follow specific points on the myocardium and track them from ED to ES. This is the idea behind the recently developed MRI tagging procedure which allows to follow a material point throughout the contraction and thus correctly determine the local myocardial function.

MRI tagging started in 1988 by Zerhouni et al.,[23] it was followed with spatial modulation of magnetization (SPAMM) by Axel et al.[47] a year later. The idea behind the tagging technique suggested by Zerhouni et al.[23] is quite ingenious: an RF pulse is applied prior to the imaging sequence to a plane perpendicular to the imaged plane. The spins in the intersection line between these two planes are "saturated", i.e., their transverse magnetization is nulled. Consequently, these lines, which represent actual material lines, appear as dark lines in the MRI image and deform as the myocardium deforms. Thus, a sequence of images at different time points along the cardiac cycle allows to visualize the patterns of the myocardial deformations. The typical radially tagged image of a human LV, depicted in Figure 8A, demonstrates how the tag lines have deformed along with the myocardium.

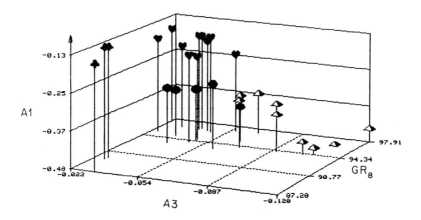

Figure 7. Representation of 27 feature vectors in the parametric space A_1–A_3–GR_8, corresponding to data obtained from a group of 27 human hearts. Note the well defined clusters formed by each group of hearts ($\heartsuit$ = Normals, $\clubsuit$ = Hypertrophic, $\bullet$ = Myocardial infarction, $\triangle$ = Aneurism) (printed with permission from Azhari et al.[46] © 1991 IEEE).

The idea behind the SPAMM technique[47] is that a magnetic gradient applied between nonselective RF pulses yields a set of dark lines separated by a distance d which depends on the magnetic gradient applied and the gyromagnetic constant. Applying two SPAMM sequences along two orthogonal directions prior to the imaging phase yields a lattice shaped tag pattern. A typical lattice configured SPAMM image of a heart is depicted in Figure 8B.

However, the 2D analysis of tagged MRI does not yield the complete picture, as the tissue may move in and out of the imaging planes due to LV longitudinal deformation and substantial twist. Thus, images acquired at different cardiac phases may correspond to different tissue segments, and techniques which account for the 3D nature of LV deformation are needed to accurately assess the patterns of myocardial strains.

Rogers et al.[48] suggested applying RF tag pulses to planes parallel to the imaged plane. A sort of a sandwich is obtained; the top and bottom planes are saturated spins that can not emit any signal during the readout phase, and the center of this sandwich is an isolated slice of the heart. The signal from this MRI sandwich images only the center plane even if parts of it will move up or down.

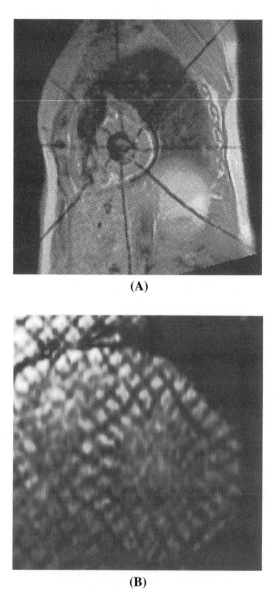

(A)

(B)

Figure 8. (A) A typical MRI image of a radially tagged heart. Note the deformation of the originally straight tag lines on the myocardium. (B) A typical SPAMM image of a heart at ES. Note the deformed lattice of tag lines which were straight and orthogonal at ED. (SPAMM Image provided courtesy of Prof. Leon Axel, University of Pennsylvania School of Medicine, USA).

The idea was further extended by Azhari et al.[49] into a "triple sandwich" whereby a tagged myocardial cuboid was isolated in space. Using a different approach, Azhari et al.[50] and Moore et al.[51] have combined information from sets of long and short axis orthogonal planes to reconstruct a set of some 24 myocardial cuboids for the canine heart, at ED and ES, and calculated the strain field for each cuboid. This technique was used by Azhari et al.,[52] for accurate mapping of ischemic regions, and, more recently by Dong et al.[53] for hypertrophic cardiomyopathy and right ventricular pressure overload.[54]

1.6. 3D DYNAMIC IMAGING

1.6.1. Visualization of 3D Dynamic Fields

Dynamic image analysis of the heart usually involves continuous smooth functions of space and time reflecting the temporal behavior of distributed parameters. *Directly measured* dynamic fields include infrared image sequences of a temperature field, or dynamic SPECT or PET tomograms which reflect changes in radioisotope concentration in specific regions of the heart. *Estimated* dynamic fields, such as 3D heart wall dynamic motion and thickness are calculated based on Cine-CT[20] or dynamic cardiac MRI[55] tomographic measurements and edge detection algorithms.[9,56−58]

The estimated instantaneous regional wall thickness H and motion magnitude M of each volume and surface elements of the myocardium can be color coded and superimposed on the 3D images of the LV. A typical color-coded 3D reconstruction of a human LV is shown in Figure 9. Abnormal wall motion is assigned a red color. A 3D wire-frame reconstruction of a human heart (Figure 10, right) and the consequent color-coded 3D wall thickening is shown in Figure 10 (left). The animated consecutive images then give a color coded 3D representation of the thickness and motion magnitude dynamics. This procedure yields a complicated 3D dynamic data set combining shape and functional information. While some general features of the shape-function relationship can be visually evident from these animated data, a considerable degree of adaptation of the human operator is needed to treat the instantaneous 3D shape and color-coded functional data simultaneously.

The great difficulty of visualization of 3D dynamic data on the 2D computer screen can be circumvented by surface mapping techniques which transform the 3D dynamic data into 2D slices at different cross-sections of the heart. The mapping procedure is based on polar unwrapping of the LV surface and representing it as a 2D bull's-eye map.[58] Three-dimensional thickness $H(r, \theta)$ and motion $M(r, \theta)$ are mapped for each angular value of θ, starting from the slice closest to the apex area, which is assigned the minimal radial

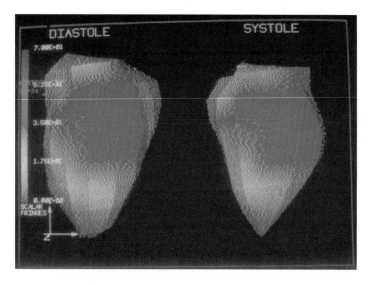

Figure 9. 3D color coded reconstructions of an abnormal human LV. Color scale corresponds to the LV wall motion values. Abnormal wall motion is assigned a red color. Note the clearly visible infarcted region. (See Color Plate I)

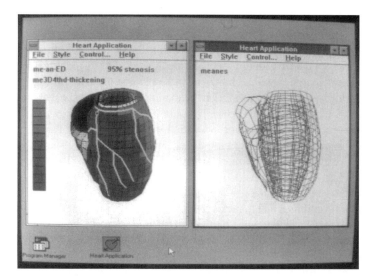

Figure 10. 3D wireframe reconstruction of a human heart (right) and its consequent color coded reconstruction depicting 3D wall thickening. Note that abnormal thickening is assigned here a blue color. (See Color Plate II)

size r, and proceeding until the last slice in the data. For simplicity, fixed angular and radial sizes of each surface element of the LV surface can be taken for each of the slices. Once the data is mapped, these 2D fields can be animated at arbitrary speeds so as to facilitate the analysis of fast dynamic changes in the image sequence. Obvious errors are due to masking of brightness variations and the nonhomogeneous background.[59]

An alternate approach is based on 2D mapping of, say, the endocardial surface and then color-coding the temporal coordinate, as for instance, the time period required to activate any point on the surface. This approach was used to map the spatio-temporal progress of the electro-activation of the myocardium.[60–62]

1.6.2. Functional Dynamic Imaging

The dynamic shape-function relationship can identify cases of early functional abnormalities in the early stage of disease development. Dynamic imaging can thus provide additional information by visualizing the precise sequence of events which may be partially abnormal, yet show normal ED to ES shape change.

Functional images generation were originated in nuclear medicine dynamic studies and a number of approaches were proposed to construct functional images.[59,63,64]

Functional images of parameters. Consider a dynamic field $H(r, \Theta, t)$ or $M(r, \Theta, t)$. For each surface element we consider it's temporal dynamics and extract spatial distribution of scalar parameters $F(r, \Theta)$, describing the dynamic process. Several examples of these parameters are: the amplitude of temporal changes, activation and relaxation time and intensity change velocity. Local motion, thickness or thickening represent some of the parameters that can be used for evaluating the LV functional dynamics. A simple functional image describing the change of thickness between the ES and ED reduces to the absolute LV thickening, similar to that described earlier.[8,10,43] However, considerable local inhomogeneity of the LV thickness can exist in some cases and it is therefore necessary to trace the relative local thickness variations rather than the absolute thickness values. This is achieved by calculating local temporal derivatives of the original image sequence. Other parametric functional images may included the speed of thickness relaxation after ES in different regions of the LV, detecting time of maximum thickening at different regions of the LV surface, and calculating maximum and minimum values of thickness and motion magnitude, etc.

Dynamic processes which are hard to describe by a single scalar parameter or by a small set of parameters can be dealt with by using specific functional imaging methods such as spatial correlation or segmentation of dynamic fields based on temporal behavior.[59,63]

1.6.3. Automatic LV Boundary Detection of Cine-CT Data

Most measurements of cardiac geometry are based on time consuming manual tracing.[3,65] The reported algorithm[56,58] for automatic identification of the endocardial and epicardial boundaries is based on the Set-Theoretic method.[66] A set of *a priori* information[56] is used to obtain a boundary estimate. It is assumed that the LV shape is rounded. The boundary lies in a specific region of the image which can be determined from the obvious anatomical structure. The heart boundaries reconstruction can simultaneously use both endocardial and epicardial data, with additional constraints on the LV wall thickness function. Wall thickness is limited by some appropriate minimum and maximum values and was assumed to be a slowly varying smooth function in the neighboring regions of the LV. The algorithm[56] is based on iterative procedures which update the boundaries estimates at each iteration step according to the imposed *a priori* information.

The algorithm was applied to Cine-CT computed tomographic data of normal and diseased heart patients obtained from the University of Iowa Hospital.[8] Contrast agent was used to increase the blood visibility. Slices were 8 mm thick; 10 images of each slice were obtained per cardiac cycle at 70 msec intervals.

The proposed method is quite successful in avoiding severe image artifacts.[56] The complete 3D dynamic Cine-CT sequence consisting of 8 spatial slices and 10 time frames for each slice is automatically traced in about 3 min on a 486 IBM compatible unit. Two-dimensional contours are estimated in 64 angular locations for each slice and time instant. Figure 11 presents an example of automatically traced temporal sequences of a single Cine-CT cross-section for a normal and an aneurysmal heart. A detailed analysis of these slices reveals a considerable number of image artifacts. These include low image contrast, noise, intensity artifacts and papillary muscles, determination of the LV boundaries.[58]

1.6.4. 3D Reconstruction of the Dynamic LV Shape

Whereas the helical 3D reconstruction procedure of Azhari *et al.*[42] allows quantitative identification of abnormal hearts and sorting them according to specific pathologies, another procedure can be used when we want to study individual hearts. The details of the 3D reconstruction and shading procedure have been described by Halmann *et al.*[10] Briefly, the detected

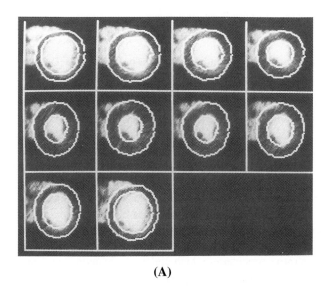

(A)

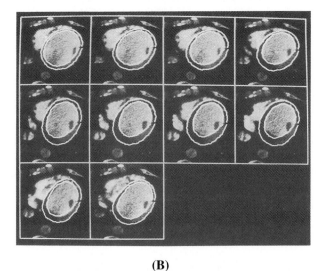

(B)

Figure 11. Results of the automatic tracing of the LV Cine-CT images (A) Tracing of a normal LV sequence (B) tracing of an abnormal LV sequence. (Reprinted from A. Taratorin and S. Sideman, *Comput. Med. Imaging and Graphics*, **19**, © 1995, 113–129, with kind permission from Elsevier Science Ltd., The Boulevard, Langford Lane, Kidlington 0X5 1GB, UK.)

2D contours representing the locations of the endocardial and epicardial boundaries of the LV are placed on top of each other, keeping the interslice gaps to obtain a 3D wireframe image. A surface element of the LV is defined by two pairs of points with similar angular locations from two consecutive slices. The resulting surface may be reconstructed from any angle of view, and rotated and shaded according to depth or gradient-shading scheme. Figure 12 presents an example of sequential wireframe reconstruction of the LV shape for a normal and an aneurysmal heart.

1.7. REGIONAL SHAPE-FUNCTION ANALYSIS

Quantification of wall motion is a "slippery ground",[5] and numerous studies dealing with regional myocardial function have been reported, with the term "function" defined somewhat arbitrarily by the many investigators. Clearly it is the movement of the endocardial wall that causes the blood to flow in the various organs in the body. However, not all types of the myocardial motion actually contribute to ejection. Furthermore, damaged tissue can be pulled by the adjacent healthy tissue and thus appear to be moving properly.

The problem stems from two sources: (1) most imaging modalities provide only 2D information while the heart is moving and contracting in 3D, and (2) it is impossible to distinguish between regional wall motion and global LV translation without following specific points on the myocardium. The last obstacle may be easily visualized by drawing two concentric circles and two eccentric circles with similar diameters. Assuming that the larger circle represents the endocardial boundary at ED and the smaller one at ES, one can estimate the corresponding wall motion for each boundary. While the concentric case yields an homogeneous pattern, the eccentric case yields an heterogeneous pattern. This is an important observation since global function, i.e., stroke volume or ejection fraction, may be identical in both these cases, while the regional wall motion differs

1.7.1. Analyses Based on Wall Motion

Two dimensional angiographic and echographic images are the most common source of information available in the clinic today, and many attempts have been made to utilize them to derive wall motion based on different spatial definitions.[5] Some have aligned the centroid points of each traced image, and some have used the LV long axis as a reference.[67] Others have tried to define a center point of contraction.[68] However, none of these 2D procedures is completely accurate.

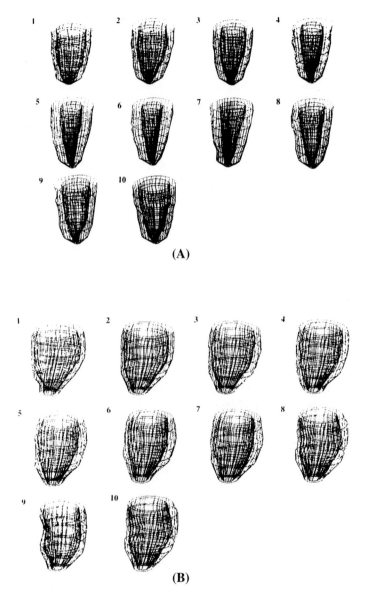

Figure 12. 3D wireframe reconstruction of the LV shape dynamics, (A) Normal LV (B) Abnormal LV. (Reprinted from A. Taratorin and S. Sideman, *Comput. Med. Imaging and Graphics*, **19**, © 1995, 113–129, with kind permission from Elsevier Science Ltd., The Boulevard, Langford Lane, Kidlington OX5 1GB, UK.)

Wall motion in the 3D domain can be determined by the difference between the average position of the four corners of the endocardial surface of a surface element at end-systole, and the corresponding surface at end-diastole, thus giving the average change in the endocardial position during contraction. Alternatively, the perpendicular motion of the endocardial surface is obtained by using three dimensional local stroke volume approach.[69] In this method, the volume which is defined by the local endocardial displacement is calculated and divided by the calculated average of the end-diastolic and end-systolic endocardial surface areas to yield the perpendicular displacement of the endocardium.

1.7.2. Analysis Based on Wall Thickness and Wall Thickening

The inability to define LV wall motion satisfactorily stimulated alternative descriptors of regional myocardial function. Beyar *et al.*[69] have proposed a 3D approach which yields a more reliable value of wall thickness. The LV wall is assumed to be made of 3D cuboids and the thickness, T, is given by:

$$T = \frac{2 \cdot V}{(A_{endo} + A_{epi})} \tag{9}$$

where, A_{endo} and A_{epi} are the cuboid's endocardial and epicardial surface areas, respectively, and V is its volume. As shown,[69] Equation (10) is valid regardless of the spatial orientation of the LV with respect to the imaging planes.

Since the myocardial mass is constant, wall thickness increases during systole in order to compensate for the reduction of the internal dimensions of the heart. This phenomenon is best characterized by relating to the wall thickening index, which is defined as the ratio of the difference between ES thickness and ED thickness to the ED thickness. As ischemic or infarcted regions cannot contract properly, their wall thickness will either remain unchanged, or even decrease if the region bulges out (e.g., in aneurysm[8]). These characteristics can help discriminate between healthy and ischemic tissue even in cases where the abnormal tissue is "pulled" by the surrounding tissue and the wall motion is apparently normal. Furthermore, thickening is insensitive to translation movements.

In order to understand the difficulty in properly defining the *wall thickness*, consider two parallel planes representing the endocardial and epicardial surfaces. If the two surfaces are not parallel, two significantly different distances will be obtained, when one measures the normals to the first or the second plane. Furthermore, typical wall thickness is about one centimeter while typical image resolution is in the order of one millimeter. Thus, any distance measured between two traced points on the myocardium will have a typical measurement error of about 10%, which in addition to image noise may prevent one from detecting mildly infarcted regions.

Lieberman et al.[70] calculated the relationship between 2D regional wall motion and thickening in myocardial infarcted dogs. Their findings have shown that wall thickness discriminates better than wall motion between the ischemic zone and the remote normal wall.

Despite its improved discriminatory potential over wall motion, 2D thickness remains an inherently limited index. Its major disadvantage stems from its inability to discriminate between wall thickness which results from tissue contraction and pseudo-wall thickness which results from the change in α, the angle of intersection between the imaging plane and the LV wall. As the imaging plane is fixed in the rooms coordinate system, the LV can move in 3D and change its orientation relative to this plane. The corresponding thickness appearing on the image plane would be:

$$T' = \frac{T_0}{\cos(90° - \alpha)} \tag{10}$$

where T' is the thickness which appears on the image plane while T_0 is the actual wall thickness. As the observed thickness is a function of α, any significant changes in the spatial orientation of the LV can yield different results.

3D motion, T_h, is similarly defined by relating to the cuboid formed in space as the endocardium moves from ED to ES. Thus,

$$T_h = \frac{2V_e}{A_{ED} - A_{ES}} \tag{11}$$

where V_e is the volume displaced by the moving endocardium (i.e., local stroke volume), and A_{ED} and A_{ES} denote the surface area of the cuboids at ED and ES, respectively.[8,12] As shown,[43] 3D wall thickening from ED to ES has an advantage over 3D motion analysis and that 3D thickening is better than 2D thickening in identifying ischemia.

Even when using this 3D approach to evaluate the regional function of the heart, the true correspondence between the ED and ES surfaces remains unsolved. For example, different material slices of the myocardium are imaged at ED and ES as the heart contracts in the longitudinal direction.[48] As a partial solution to this problem, Azhari et al.[7] have suggested to use the helical coordinate system which contracts longitudinally along with the heart. This assures some degree of tissue tracking in the longitudinal direction and myocardial tissue segments sampled at ED will be closely related to those selected at ES. Using this approach on MRI and post mortem data, Azhari et al.[12] have shown that ischemic myocardial regions can be identified with an overall accuracy of about 74%. Furthermore, they have shown that 3D thickness analysis is superior to 3D wall motion analysis.

1.7.3. Strain Analysis

The systolic strain field provides another vehicle which can be used to describe the regional left or right ventricular function.[52] Many investigators have attempted to measure the strain field with or without associated imaging procedures. For example, Prinzen et al.[71] have employed needles which were inserted into the LV wall and measured the shortening of the inner myocardial layers. Dieudonne[72] and others have sewed strain gauges to the myocardium. Hawthorne et al.[73] have sewed mercury filled rubber tubes to the myocardium and measured its deformations by studying the changes in their electrical resistance. Waldman et al.[74] and others have implanted many a small metal beads into the myocardium of canine hearts. The beads were tracked using biplannar angiographic studies, and the regional strain tensor was calculated from their deformations. Yun et al.[75] and others have inserted small metal screws into the myocardium of human hearts. The corresponding myocardial deformations were evaluated by tracking the metal screws with biplannar angiography.

Freeman et al.,[76] Villarell et al.[77] and many others have inserted pairs of miniature ultrasonic transducers into the myocardium in order to measure regional deformations. Others (Prinzen et al.[78]) suggested the use of small optical markers which were glued to the epicardium and tripodal strain gauge devices attached by suction to the epicardium (e.g., Lab et al.[79]) to study epicardial strains. All the above mentioned techniques suffer from the same disadvantages: they are invasive in nature, requiring surgical procedures which may affect the studied tissue and the consequent results.

While all these invasive studies provide important physiological data, they are nevertheless unsuitable for clinical practice. The recent developments of non-invasive imaging techniques, and particular MRI tagging now allow to determine realistic nonhomogeneous regional movement and local strain/stress characteristics.[50,52]

1.7.4. Regional Stress Indices

Local average circumferential and meridional σ/P can be approximated by the following Janz equations:[80]

$$(\sigma/P)_c = r_c r_m [2 - r_c/r_m \sin\phi]/[2t \sin\phi(r_m + t/2)] \tag{12}$$

$$(\sigma/P)_m = r_c^2/[2t \sin\phi(r + t \sin\phi/2)] \tag{13}$$

Table 1. Global parameters of normal left ventricles ($n = 9$).

Parameter	Unit	Mean
ED Volume	ml	143.3 ± 21.9
ES Volume	ml	43.0 ± 10.3
Stroke Volume	ml	100.3 ± 14.7
EF	%	70.1 ± 4.0
ED Mass	g	140.6 ± 18.8
ES Mass	g	141.1 ± 23.4
ED Surface		
Endo	cm^2	135.9 ± 11.9
Epi	cm^2	195.5 ± 16.6
ES Surface		
Endo	cm^2	70.5 ± 10.4
Epi	cm^2	149.9 ± 16.0
Endo Change	%	48.3 ± 4.4
Epi Change	%	23.8 ± 3.1

where subscripts c and m denote circumferential and meridional components, respectively, r is the radius of curvature, ϕ is the angle between the normal to the endocardium and the left ventricular long axis and t is the wall thickness.

Equations (12) and (13) are based on the thick-wall shell theory, assuming symmetry about the axis, absence of shear stresses and constant wall thickness. However, the equations have the advantage of being more applicable to a general representation of ventricular geometry than a sphere, cylinder or ellipsoid, and may therefore be used to account for the irregular shapes which occur in both normal and diseased LVs.[8,81]

1.8. SHAPE-FUNCTION CHARACTERISTICS OF THE NORMAL HEART

Left ventricular volumes, mass, stroke volume, ejection fraction, and endocardial and epicardial surface areas for a group of 9 normal volunteers are summarized in Table 1. Longitudinal shortening averaged $16.7 \pm 3.9\%$.[81]

Wall thickness. Average wall thickness increases from 0.89 ± 0.05 cm at end-diastole to 1.44 ± 0.07 cm at end-systole. Circumferentially, thickness is smallest anteriorly at end-diastole, while at end-systole the lateral wall is significantly larger ($p < 0.01$). End-diastolic wall thickness increases gradually from apex to base. End-systolic thickness increases up to approximately two-thirds of the way between apex and base, and then decreases gradually towards the base.[81]

Wall thickening. Wall thickening averages $66 \pm 12\%$ globally. The highest values are at the lateral wall ($82 \pm 17\%$, $p < 0.01$) and the smallest values are at the septum ($46 \pm 8\%$, $p < 0.01$). Thickening in the longitudinal direction decreases from $72 \pm 16\%$ near the apex to $49 \pm 15\%$ towards the base.[81]

Wall motion. Wall motion, determined as the displacement of the endocardial surface element from ED to its corresponding location at ES, is compared to the 3D stroke-volume-element approach which yields the motion perpendicular to the wall. The results of the volume element approach are uniformly some 15% smaller than those calculated by planar displacement, but the regional variation displayed a similar pattern in both these methods. Data show that wall motion is smallest at the septum (5.9 ± 1.6 mm) increasing anteriorly and posteriorly, and largest laterally (11.2 ± 1.7 mm).[81]

Stress/pressure index. The stress/pressure index (σ/P) is relatively evenly distributed, circumferentially and meridionally in the LV, i.e. the standard deviations are relatively small considering the number of parameters involved in their estimation. Nevertheless, regional differences in stress/pressure (σ/P) index are evident; circumferential values are in all cases significantly larger at the septum ($p < 0.01$). Longitudinally, there is a small gradual moderate increase in both circumferential and meridional σ/P from apex to base at both ED and ES.[81]

1.9. COMPARISON OF DYNAMIC LV MOTION AND THICKNESS OF NORMAL AND ANEURYSMAL HEARTS

Dynamic 3D geometry of the LV. Visual comparison of the sequence of 3D wireframe images of normal and aneurysmal hearts presented in Figure 12 reveals several obvious differences. The contraction and relaxation of the normal LV looks homogenous both at the septal area (left side of the wireframe image) and at the free wall (right side of the wireframe). End-systole takes place approximately in the middle of the cardiac cycle; the contraction and relaxation phases are symmetric as judged by motion dynamics (Figure 12). The aneurysmal LV is characterized by a non-dynamic thin LV wall in the septal region (left side of the wireframe images). Reasonable thickening occurs only in the region of free wall and the ES state is late (frame 8) and is followed by fast relaxation of the free wall thickness. The aneurysmal region is bent inside the LV cavity during this fast relaxation phase (frames 8, 9), probably due to the sharp fall of the LV cavity pressure compared to the right ventricle (RV).

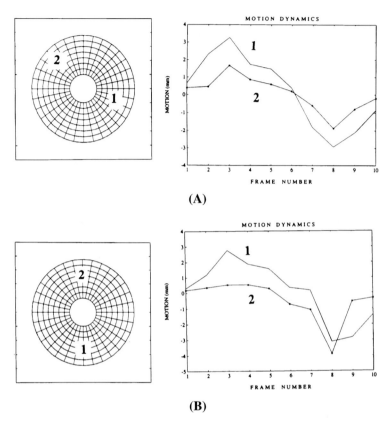

Figure 13. Graphs of motion magnitude dynamics in two selected regions of interest; (A) Normal heart (1–free wall, 2–septum). (B) Aneurysmal heart (1–normal region, 2–aneurysmal region). (Reprinted from A. Taratorin and S. Sideman, *Comput. Med. Imaging and Graphics*, **19**, © 1995, 113–129, with kind permission from Elsevier Science Ltd., The Boulevard, Langford Lane, Kidlington 0X5 1GB, UK.)

Dynamic motion magnitude variations. The sequence of polar maps of absolute regional instantaneous endocardium motion magnitude[58,82] is represented here by the corresponding temporal graphs for the normal and aneurysmal LVs (Figure 13). Motion dynamics of the normal LV is characterized by the movement of the LV endocardium "into" the LV cavity during contraction and the symmetric expansion of the LV during relaxation (curve 1). Inhomogeneity of the endocardial motion is noticed in the septal region and a delay in the onset of contraction and relaxation (curve 2), which is approximately equal to 100 ms. The distribution of instantaneous endocardial motion magnitude of the aneurysmal LV is radically different from the normal case. The aneurysmal region does not move significantly during the contraction phase (curve 1) and experiences strong movement into the LV cavity during relaxation. Distant normal endocardial regions are characterized by moderate motion inside the LV cavity during contraction and strong outside motion during the relaxation, similar to that in the aneurysmal area (curve 2).

Dynamic thickness variations. The sequence of the polar thickness maps for the normal LV[58] shows that the thickness dynamics is practically homogenous in the different LV regions. A similar sequence of maps for the aneurysmal LV is asymmetric.[58] The corresponding time courses of thickness in selected ROI, presented in Figure 14, show that the myocardial thickness is identical everywhere in the normal LV, and differs significantly in the aneurysmal hearts. The dynamics of the remote normal region thickness (curve 2), are asymmetric, describing prolonged contraction and fast relaxation of this region of the diseased LV. Similarly, the "border zone"[8] lying between the aneurysmal and distant normal LV regions is characterized by reduced myocardial function.

Functional images of 3D thickness and motion dynamics. An integral representation of the information contained in the sequences of the polar maps of LV thickness and motion can be obtained by using functional images of the 3D LV based on the reconstructed ED and ES. These include the parametric 3D functional images color-coded to describe the magnitude of thickness changes for the normal and pathological hearts.[8,12,58,82] Other presentations include the images of spatially correlated dynamics for the heart. Note that the normal LV is again characterized by a monogenous temporal dynamics of thickness while the aneurysmal heart is characterized by several distinct spatial regions of the LV representing different dynamic thickness behaviors from ED to ES. The dynamic segmentation method applied to the aneurysmal LV based on wall thickness results in distinct segmentation between different regions.

Functional images can also demonstrate the spatial distribution of the ratio of thickening to thinning rate. It can be seen[58] that this ratio is homogenous for the normal LV while it is asymmetric for the aneurysmal LV, marking the fast relaxation rate in the distant normal LV regions in the myocardium.

1.10. VENTRICULAR INTERACTION AND REGIONAL FUNCTION

While most imaging efforts have concentrated on the LV, some studies deal with the effect of pathology in one ventricle on the shape-function relationship of the other.

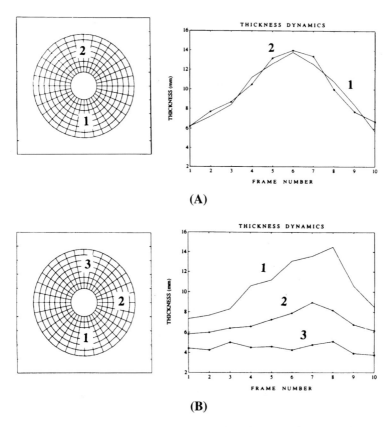

Figure 14. Graphs of thickness dynamics in selected regions of interest; (A) Normal heart. (B) Aneurysmal heart (1–normal region, 2–transient region, 3–aneurysmal region). (Reprinted from A. Taratorin and S. Sideman, *Comput. Med. Imaging and Graphics*, **19**, © 1995, 113–129, with kind permission from Elsevier Science Ltd., The Boulevard, Langford Lane, Kidlington 0X5 1GB, UK.)

Since the ventricular septum is common to the LV and RV, the LV shape is distorted in acute and chronic RV pressure overload (RVPO) by the flattening, or leftward displacement, of the septum.[54,83–87] Since the septum is common to both the LV and the RV, RVPO and septal flattening is accompanied by changes in the LV regional systolic function. Thus, acute RVPO, which is induced by pulmonary arterial constriction, leads to a decrease in LV regional ED segment length as well as to a decrease in systolic segment shortening of the septum and the free wall;[88,89] these segmental changes are heterogeneously distributed circumferentially[88,89] and transmurally.[90]

Using tagged MRI technique, 3D reconstruction, and the volume element approach, Dong *et al.*[54] reported systolic global and regional LV performance in relation to the distortion of the LV cross-sectional shape and the severity of the disease. It is interesting to note that while the LV was distorted in both diastole and systole due to the RV pathology, the overall ventricular performance was preserved, despite the reduced septal myocardial performance (as assessed by systolic wall thickening and segment shortening). The consequent LV shape changes involved a decrease in the circumferential shortening in the septal and lateral walls; the magnitude of this decrease was closely related to the degree of LV distortion. Global LV function was maintained even in seven cases of RVPO with reduced myocardial performance. This was manifested by a bellows-like systolic motion of the septum and the LV free wall relative to each other.

The inverse effect of LV pathology on the RV shape-function relationship has been demonstrated by Guez *et al.*[91] The study deals with the 3D analysis of the effect of LV aneurysm on the regional RV shape-function (wall motion) relationship. Using Cine-CT data, Guez *et al.*[91] used the 3D stroke volume element approach to determine the endocardial RV wall motion. Analysis of Cine-CT data from 9 normal hearts and 10 hearts of patients with aneurysms showed that a higher posterior than anterior endocardial motion characterizes both groups. No longitudinal variations in motion were found in the normal hearts. However, the study shows that endocardial motion of the RV is affected by LV aneurysm, mostly by a change in the longitudinal variations of wall motion manifested by increased basal motion and decreased apical motion.

1.11. DISCUSSION

Cardiac imaging typically provides information on the instantaneous geometry of the heart. Most studies to date have extracted clinical information from cardiac images by analyzing the temporal changes of desired geometrical features such as wall motion, thickness, thickening, and strain. Furthermore, most studies have related only to the 2D information available from cross-sectioned images.

A more comprehensive approach which accounts for the 3D nature of the problem is presented here. Information of clinical merit can be extracted from the changes in the shape of the hearts as well as from its instantaneous geometry. The unique properties of the geometrical cardiogram (GCG) allow to quantify the LV 3D shape. By applying Fourier and KLT transforms to the GCG, it is possible to determine abnormality and sort the heart's pathology by studying the 3D shape.

The combination of dynamic 3D LV shape animation, temporal study of the LV thickness and motion and functional imaging presents a number of possibilities for the characterization of the *shape-function* relationship of the LV. In the particular case of fibrous aneurysms, the differences between the normal and aneurysmal LV dynamics are distinct. While the integrated 3D ED to ES variations of motion and thickness provide very significant functional information, important observations were obtained for the dynamic changes in LV geometry. Specifically, prolonged thickening and fast thickness relaxation was demonstrated in the normal regions of the aneurysmal LV.[58] This effect was theoretically predicted in a number of studies.[92] While these findings are yet to be validated by additional data, they demonstrate the importance of detailed dynamic analysis tools for cardiac studies. Thickness, motion and stress and strain information are undoubtedly helpful in the detailed characterization of the LV dynamics.

It has been suggested that the thickness variations are more reliable for the characterization of regional myocardial function.[20,58] This is primarily due to the fact that motion magnitude changes might be influenced not only by the local cardiac muscle activity but by the overall movement of the heart and different mechanical interactions. Tagging, together with 3D reconstruction,[50–52,93] presents a most powerful tool whereby the problems of translation and rotation of material with elements at different phases of the cardiac cycle can be solved to yield an ultimate "gold standard" method of measurement.

1.12. CONCLUSION

The importance of accurate measurement of cardiac shape and dynamics can not be overemphasized, as it reflects a scope of cardiac diseases which are the major cause of mortality in developed countries today. Cardiac imaging plays the major role in regard, and almost the only one in this clinical context.

This chapter describes a number of methodologies for the detailed analysis of LV geometry using data obtained from various imaging modalities (ultrasound, CT, MRI). The 3D LV shape can be quantitatively characterized and analyzed by combining the methods of 3D reconstruction with the GCG shape descriptor. LV function can be quantified by calculating regional wall thickness, wall motion, radius of curvature or myocardial strains, and their spatio-temporal analysis. A number of new dynamic effects are described for both normal and abnormal LVs. It is demonstrated herein that automatic geometry based sorting of normal and abnormal hearts is feasible and that accurate definition of an aneurysmal LV region is possible in a variety of ways. Future research will extend applications of the proposed methods to the analysis of other cardiac pathologies and will lead to better understanding of the dynamic *shape-function* relationship of the LV.

Obviously, many other important studies related to cardiac analysis and medical imaging, namely the use of PET and SPECT, the use of MRI contrast agents and the use of MRI spectroscopy, all of which deserve special attention, are not included in this chapter.

1.13. ACKNOWLEDGEMENTS

This study was sponsored by the Women's Division of the American Technion Society, New York, USA. We acknowledge with particular appreciation the personal grants from Rose and Ervine Seidman, NY, USA, Mr. Yochai Schneider, Las Vegas, USA and Mr. David Salzberg, Florida, USA. Thanks are due to Dr. Mel Marcus (deceased) and Dr. William Stanford of the University of Iowa Hospital for making these cardiac images available. We also wish to acknowledge the help of the Edith and Joseph Jackier, Al and Phyllis Newman (Detroit, MI, USA) and the Michal and Adelaide Kennedy-Leigh (London, UK) endowment funds.

1.14. REFERENCES

1. Mirsky, I., D.N. Ghista and H. Sandler, 1974, *Cardiac Mechanics* (John Wiley & Sons, Inc., Canada).
2. Pohost, G.M. and R.A. O'Rourke (eds.), 1991, *Principles and Practice of Cardiovascular Imaging* (Little, Brown & Company, Boston).
3. Marcus, M.L., W. Stanford, Z. Hajduczo and R.M. Weiss, 1989, *Am. J. Cardiol.*, **64**, E54–E59.
4. Collins, S. and D. Skorton, 1986, *Cardiac Imaging and Image Processing* (McGraw Hill, New York).
5. Sigwart, U. and P.H. Heintzen (eds.), 1984, *Ventricular Wall Motion* (Georg Thieme Verlag, Stuttgart).
6. Hoffman, E.A., 1991, in: *3D Imaging in Medicine* (J.K. Udupa and G.T. Herman, eds.) (CRC Press, Boca Raton, FL) pp. 285–311.
7. Azhari, H., R. Beyar, E. Grenadier, U. Dinnar and S. Sideman, 1987, *IEEE Trans. Biomed. Eng.*, **34**, 345–355.
8. Lessick, J., S. Sideman, H. Azhari, M. Marcus, E. Grenadier and R. Beyar, 1991, *Circulation*, **84**(3), 1072–1086.
9. Wang, J., R. Mezrich and W. Welkowitz, 1990, in: *Imaging, Analysis and Simulation of the Cardiac System* (S. Sideman and R. Beyar, eds.) (Freund Publ. House, London), pp. 35–53.
10. Halmann, M., S. Sideman, H. Azhari, W. Markiewicz and R. Beyar, 1990, *Basic Res. Cardiol.*, **85**, 429–434.
11. Sideman, S., R. Beyar, H. Azhari, E. Barta, D. Adam and U. Dinnar, 1988, *IEEE Proc*, 76/6, 708–719.
12. Azhari, H., R. Beyar and S. Sideman, 1990, in: *Imaging, Analysis and Simulation of the Cardiac System* (S. Sideman and R. Beyar, eds.) (Freund Publ. House, London) pp. 105–126.
13. Gibson, D., 1990, in: *Imaging, Analysis and Simulation of the Cardiac System* (S. Sideman and R. Beyar, eds.) (Freund Publ. House, London) pp. 89–103.

14. Duncan, J., L. Staib and A. Amini, 1991, *Proc. IEEE Eng. Med. & Biol. Ann. Conf.*, **13**, 287–288.

15. Frossman, W., 1974, *Klin. Wochenscho*, **8**(1929), 2085; in: *Cardiac Catheterization and Angioplasty* (W. Grossman, ed.), (Leal & Feiger, Philadelphia), p. 4.

16. Hisagana, K. and A. Hisagana, 1978, *Ultrasound in Medicine* (D. White and E.A. Lyons, eds.) (Plenum Press, NY), **4**, pp. 391–402.

17. Nakamura, S., D.J. Mahon, B. Maheswaran, D.E. Gutfinger, A. Colombo and J.M. Tobis, 1995, *J. Am. Coll. Cardiol.*, **25**, 633–639.

18. Schelbert, H.R., 1993, in: *Imaging in Transport Processes* (S. Sideman and K. Hijikata, eds.), (Begell House Publ., NY), pp. 577–586.

19. Robb, R.A., E.A. Hoffman, L.J. Sinak, L.D. Harris and E.L. Ritman, 1983, *Proc. IEEE*, **71**, 308–319.

20. Collins, S.M., P. Yashodar, J.A. Rumberger, A.J. Feiring, M.P. Noel, K.B. Chandran, S.R. Fleagle, M.L. Marcus and D.J. Skorton, 1985, *Proc. Comp. in Cardiol.*, **12**, 67–72.

21. Mansfield, P., P.G. Morris and J.S. Waugh (eds.), 1982, *Advances in Magnetic Resonance* (Academic Press Inc.), Supplement 2, pp. 143–154.

22. Meyer, C.H., B.S. Hu, D.G. Nishimura and A. Macovski, 1992, *Magnetic Resonance in Med.*, **28**, 202–213.

23. Zerhouni, E.A., D.M. Parrish, W.J. Rogers, A. Yang and E.P. Shapiro, 1989, *Radiology*, **16**, 59–63.

24. Weisfeldt, M.L., R. Beyar, E.J. Shapiro, J.L. Weiss, W. Rogers and E.A. Zerhouni, 1990, in: *Imaging Analysis and Simulation of the Cardiac System* (S. Sideman and R. Beyar, eds.) (Freund Publ. House, London), pp. 3–17.

25. Grenadier, E., H. Azhari, R. Beyar, U. Dinnar, W. Markiewicz and S. Sideman, 1989, *J. Cardiovasc. Tech.*, **8**, 5–14.

26. Moritz, W.E., A.S. Pearlman, D.H. McCabe, D.K. Medema, M.E. Ainsworth and M.S. Boles, 1983, *IEEE Trans. Biomed. Eng.*, BME-30, 482–492.

27. Nixon, J.V., S.I. Saffer, K. Lipscomb and C.G. Blomqvist, 1983, *Am. Heart J.*, **106**, 435–443.

28. Woods, R.H., 1892, *J. Anat. Physiol.*, **26**, 362–370.

29. Burch, G.E., C.T. Ray and M.S. Cornvick, 1952, *Circulation*, **5**, 504–513.

30. Burton, A.C., 1957, *Am. Heart J.*, **54**, 801–810.

31. Hutchins, G.M., B.H. Bulkley, G.W. Moore, M.A. Piasio and F.T. Lohr, 1978, *Am. J. Cardiol.*, **41**, 646–654.

32. Silverman, K.J., G.M. Hutchins, J.L. Weiss and G.W. Moore, 1982, *Am. J. Cardiol.*, **49**, 27–32.

33. Gibson, D.G. and D.J. Brown, 1975, *Br. Heart J.*, **37**, 904–910.

34. Fischl, S.J., R. Gorlin and M.V. Herman, 1977, *Am. J. Cardiol.*, **39**, 170–176.

35. Azancot, A., T.P. Caudell, H.D. Allen, S. Horowitz, D.J. Sahn, C. Stoll, C. Thies, L.M. Valdex-Cruz and S.J. Goldberg, 1983, *Circulation*, **68**, 1201–1211.

36. Kass, D.A., T.A. Traill, M. Keating, P.I. Altieri and W.L. Maughan, 1988, *Circ. Res.*, **62**, 127–138.

37. Duvernoy, J., A. Jouan, J.C. Cardot, M. Baud, J. Verdenet and R. Bidet, 1986, in: *Information Processing in Medical Imaging* (Martinus Nijhoff Publishers: Dordrecht), pp. 216–222.

38. Marcus, E., P. Lorente, E. Barta, R. Beyar, D. Adam and S. Sideman, 1985, *Computers in Cardiology* (IEEE Computer Society Press/Maryland) **12**, 145–148.

39. Walley, R., M. Grover, G.L. Raff, J.W. Benge, B. Hannaford and S.A. Glantz, 1982, *Circ. Res.*, **50**, 573–589.

40. Janicki, J.S., K.T. Weber, R.F. Gochman, S. Shroff and F.J. Geheb, 1981, *Am. J. Physiol.*, **241**, H1–H11.

41. Schudy, R.B., 1979, *Proc. IEEE Workshop on Computers*, pp. 87–89.

42. Azhari, H., S. Sideman, R. Beyar, E. Grenadier and U. Dinnar, 1987, *IEEE Trans. Biomed. Eng.*, **34**, 345–355.

43. Azhari, H., S. Sideman, J.L. Weiss, E.P. Shapiro, M.L. Weisfeldt, W.L. Graves, W.J. Rogers and R. Beyar, 1990, *Am. J. Physiol.*, **259**, H1492–H1503.
44. Azhari, H., E. Grenadier, U. Dinnar, R. Beyar, D. Adam, M.L. Marcus and S. Sideman, 1989, *IEEE Trans. Biomed. Eng.*, **36**, 322–332.
45. Azhari, H., R. Beyar, M.L. Marcus and S. Sideman, 1990, *Proc. 12th Annual Int. Conf. IEEE Eng. Med. and Biology Soc.*, **12**, 230–331.
46. Azhari, H., I. Gath, R. Beyar, M.L. Marcus and S. Sideman, 1991, *IEEE Trans. Medical Imaging*, **10**, 207–215.
47. Axel, L. and L. Dougherty, 1989, *Radiology*, **171**, 841–845.
48. Rogers, W.J., E.P. Shapiro, J.L. Weiss, M.B. Buchalter, F.E. Rademaker, M.L. Weisfeldt and E.A. Zerhouni, 1991, *Circulation*, **84**, 721–731.
49. Azhari, H., W.J. Rogers, E.A. Zerhouni, J.L. Weiss, M.L. Weisfeldt and E.P. Shapiro, 1991, *Proc. Soc. of Magnetic Resonance in Medicine (SMRM)*, San Francisco, CA, Aug. 10–16, **2**, 864.
50. Azhari, H., J.L. Weiss, W.J. Rogers, C.O. Siu, E.A. Zerhouni and E.P. Shapiro, 1993, *Am. J. Physiol.*, (*Heart Circ. Physiol.*, **33**) **264**, H205–H216.
51. Moore, C.C., W.G. O'Dell, E.R. McVeigh and E.A. Zerhouni, 1992, *J. Magnet. Reson. Imag.*, **2**, 165–175.
52. Azhari, H., J.L. Weiss, W.J. Rogers, C.O. Siu and E.P. Shapiro, 1995, *Am. J. Physiol.*, (*Heart Circ. Physiol.*, **37**) **268**, H1918–H1926.
53. Dong, S.-J., J.H. MacGregor, A.P. Crawley, E. McVeigh, I. Belenkie, E.R. Smith, J.V. Tyberg and R. Beyar, 1994, *Circulation*, **90**, 1200–1209.
54. Dong, S.-J., A.P. Crawley, J.H. MacGregor, Y.F. Petrank, D.W. Bergman, I. Belenkie, E.R. Smith, J.V. Tyberg and R. Beyar, 1995, *Circulation*, **91**, 2359–2370.
55. Herfkens, R.J., 1990, in: *Imaging, Analysis and Simulation of the Cardiac System* (S. Sideman and R. Beyar, eds.), (Freund Publ. House, London), pp. 19–34.
56. Taratorin, A. and S. Sideman, 1993, *IEEE Trans. Med. Imaging*, **12**, 521–533.
57. Duncan, J., L. Staib and A. Amini, 1991, *Proc. IEEE Eng. in Med. & Bio. Ann. Conf.*, **13**, 287–288.
58. Taratorin, A. and S. Sideman, 1995, *Comput. Med. Imaging & Graphics*, **19**, 113–129.
59. Taratorin, A. and S. Sideman, 1993, in: *Imaging in Transport Processes*, S. Sideman and J. Hijikata (eds.) (Begell House, NY), pp. 21–30.
60. Barta, E., D. Adam, E. Salant and S. Sideman, 1987, *Annals Biomed. Eng.*, **15**, 443–456.
61. Barta, E. and S. Sideman, 1988, *Computers in Cardiology*, Belgium, Sept, 1987 (K.L. Ripley, (ed.), Computer Society Press, Washington, D.C.), pp. 495–498.
62. Barta, E. and S. Sideman, 1990, *Computers in Cardiology* (Jerusalem, Sept. 1989), **16**, 127–130.
63. Taratorin, A. and A. Kogan, 1988, *Rep. USSR Academy of Sci.*, **298**, 560–564 (in Russian).
64. Spiesberger, W. and M. Tasto, 1981, in: *Image Sequence Analysis*, T.S. Huang (ed.), (Springer Series in Information Sciences, Vol. 5, Springer-Verlag).
65. Pohost, G.M. and R.A. O'Rourke (eds.), 1991, *Principles and Practice of Cardiovascular Imaging* (Little, Brown & Company: Boston).
66. Hurt, N.E., 1989, *Phase Retrieval and Zero Crossings: Mathematical Methods in Image Reconstruction* (Kluwer Academic Publishers: Dordrecht).
67. Lorente, P., I. Azancot, C. Maxquet, J.L. Adda, R. Saumont and R. Slama, 1984, *Biorheology*, Supp I, 175–182.
68. Moynihan, P.F., A.F. Parisi and C.L. Feldman, 1981, *Circulation*, **63**, 752–760.
69. Beyar, R., E.P. Shapiro, W.L. Graves, W.J. Rogers, W.H. Guier, G.A. Carey, R.L. Soulen, E.A. Zerhouni, M.L. Weisfeldt and J.L. Weiss, 1990, *Circulation*, **81**, 297–307.
70. Liberman, A.N., J.L. Weiss, B.I. Jugdutt, L.C. Becker and M.L. Weisfeldt, 1981, *Circulation*, **63**, 739–846.
71. Prinzen, F.W., T. Arts, G.J. Van Der Vus and R.S. Reneman, 1984, *J. Biomech.*, **17**, 801–811.
72. Dieudonne, J.M., 1969, *J. Physiol. (Paris)*, **61**, 305–330.
73. Hawthorne, E.W., 1966, *Am. J. Cardiol.*, **18**, 566–573.

74. Waldman, L.K., Y.C. Fung and J.W. Covell, 1985, *Circ. Res.*, **57**, 152–163.
75. Yun, K.L., M.A. Niczyporuk, G.T. Daughters, N.B. Ingels, E.B. Stinson, E.L. Alderman, D.E. Hansen and D.C. Miller, 1991, *Circulation*, **83**, 962–973.
76. Freeman, G.L., M.M. LeWinter, R.L. Engler and J.W. Covell, 1985, *Circ. Res.*, **56**, 31–39.
77. Villarreal, F.J. and W.Y. Lew, 1990, *Am. J. Physiol.*, (*Heart Circ. Physiol.*, **28**), **259**, H1409–1418.
78. Prinzen, F.W., C.H. Augustijn, T. Arts, M.A. Allessie and R.S. Reneman, 1990, *Am. J. Physiol.*, (*Heart Circ. Physiol.*) **259**, H300–H308.
79. Lab, M.J. and K.V. Woollard, 1978, *Cardiovasc. Res.*, **12**, 555–565.
80. Janz, R.F. and R.J. Waldron, 1978, *Circ. Res.*, **42**, 255–263.
81. Lessick, J., Y. Fisher, M. Marcus, R. Beyar, S. Sideman and H. Azhari, 1995, submitted.
82. Taratorin, A. and S. Sideman, 1994, *SPIE*, **1905**, 294–306.
83. Dong, S.-J., E.R. Smith and J.V. Tyberg, 1992, *Circulation*, **86**, 1280–1290.
84. Smith, E.R. and J.V. Tyberg, 1987, in: *Mechanics of the Circulation* (Martinus Nijhoff Publishers, Dordrecht, The Netherlands), pp. 171–188.
85. Ryan, T., O. Petrovic, J.C. Dillon, H. Feigenbaum, M.J. Conley and W.F. Armstrong, 1985, *J. Am. Coll. Cardiol.*, **5**, 918–924.
86. Ascah, K.J., M.E. King, L.D. Gillam and A.E. Weyman, 1990, *Can. J. Cardiol.*, **6**, 99–106.
87. Louie, E.K., S. Rich, S. Levitsky and B.H. Brundage, 1992, *J. Am. Coll. Cardiol.*, **19**, 84–90.
88. Molaug, M., O. Stokland, A. Ilebekk, J. Lekven and F. Kiil, 1981, *Circ. Res.*, **49**, 52–61.
89. Goto, Y., B.K. Slinker and M.M. LeWinter, 1989, *Circ. Res.*, **65**, 43–54.
90. Beyar, R., S.-J. Dong, E.R. Smith, I. Belenkie and J.V. Tyberg, 1993, *Am. J. Physiol.*, **265**, H2044–H2056.
91. Guez, D.H., S. Sideman and R. Beyar, 1994, *Third Asian Symp. on Visualization*, Chiba, Japan, May, pp. 815–820.
92. Lawrence, W.E., W.L. Maughan and D.A. Kass, 1992, *Circulation*, **82**, 816–827.
93. Young, A.A. and L. Axel, 1992, *Radiology*, **185**, 241–247.

2 TECHNIQUES IN THE ASSESSMENT OF THE LEFT VENTRICULAR FUNCTION

Abd–El–OUAHAB BOUDRAA*

Faculté de Médecine Alexis Carrel, Lyon, France
Institut de Physique de Constantine, Algérie

2.1. THE CARDIAC PUMP

The heart is a muscular pump that functions by periodic changes of shape caused by stresses induced by the myocardial fibers. It provides by far the greatest part of the force required for the blood circulation. It is very roughly conical in form. The organ consists of right and left channels. Each consists of two chambers, a thin-walled atrium behind, which receives blood through veins and a comparatively thick-walled ventricle in front, which delivers blood into a large artery arising from its upper posterior part. The posterior part of the septum separates the two atria and is called the interatrial septum, while the anterior part intervenes mainly between the two ventricles and is called the interventricular septum (Figure 1). The Left Ventricle (LV) extends from the Atrioventricular (AV) orifice, forwards, downwards, and to the apex of the heart (Figure 2). Because the peripheral resistance offered by the systemic circulation is considerably greater than that of the pulmonary circulation, its wall is some three times as thick as the Right Ventricle (RV). The thickness of the interventricular septum corresponds to that of the other left ventricular walls. It bulges markedly towards the right and consequently

---

*Present address: Faculté de Médecine Alexis Carrel, Laboratoire de Biophysique, Groupe de Recherche en Imagerie et Spectroscopie Nucléaire (EA 640). rue Guillaume Paradin, 69372 Lyon Cedex 08, France.

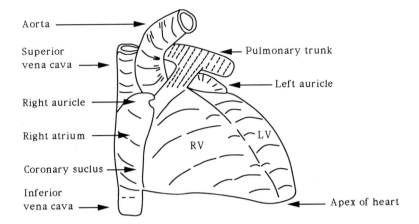

Figure 1. The external form of the heart (sternocostal surface).

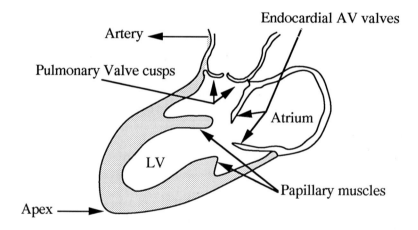

Figure 2. Heart valves in ventricular diastole.

the lumen of the LV is approximately circular in cross-section (Figure 3). The RV lumen is crescenic in cross-section (Figure 3) and RV is shorter so that its anterior part does not reach the apex of the heart (Figure 1).

During blood circulation, the right atrium receives deoxygenated blood from the systemic circulation through three veins: the superior vena cava carrying blood from the upper part of the body, the inferior vena cava draining the abdomen and the lower limbs, and the coronary sinus draining the

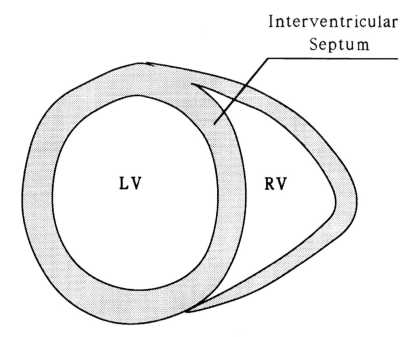

Figure 3. Vertical section of the heart.

heart itself. The blood then passed successively through the right AV orifice, the RV, and the pulmonary orifice and is carried by the pulmonary trunk and the two pulmonary arteries to the pulmonary circulation. The blood takes up oxygen from, and gives up carbon dioxide to, the air within the alveoli of the lungs, and returns to the left atrium through the two pulmonary veins on each side. After passing successively through the left AV orifice, the LV and the aortic orifice, it is carried into the systemic circulation once again through the aorta.

The cardiac cycle involves successive periods of contraction (systole) and relaxation (diastole) of the cardiac muscle. During ventricular systole, the rising pressures in the chambers first close the AV valves. Soon afterwards, the interventricular pressures reach sufficient levels to open the aortic and pulmonary valves, and the ventricles empty their blood into the arteries, the pulse expanding the elastic arterial walls. Meanwhile, the atria in diastole are passively filled with blood flowing into them from the veins. As the ventricles pass into diastole, their internal pressures fall sharply, and the elastic recoil of the arterial walls forces blood back towards the ventricles

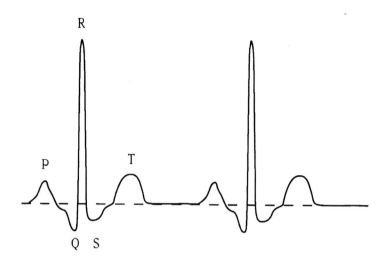

Figure 4. Electrocardiogram signal.

and closes the aortic and pulmonary valves. As ventricular diastole continues, the atria are also still in diastole. Blood from the full atria opens the AV valves and passes through the AV orifices into the ventricles. When the greatest part of the atrial contents has passed passively into the ventricles in this way, the transfer is completed and the ventricles are fully filled by a short atrial systole. Atrial systole is followed after a short interval by a ventricular systole and the cycle is repeated.

The electrical changes occuring in the myocardium during each cardiac cycle are represented by a signal known as an electrocardiogram. This normally, consists of a regular repetition of a number of waves and peaks (Figure 4). The P wave represents atrial systole and the QRS complex the slightly asynchronous contractions of different parts of the ventricles. The T wave reflects the repolarisation of the ventricular muscle. The duration of the P-R interval is a measure of the time taken for the impulse to pass over the atria and along the AV conducting tissue. The interval between the end of the S wave and the beginning of the T wave corresponds closely to the period of maximal ejection during ventricular systole.

The performance of the heart is measured by its capacity to eject, at each systolic phase, the blood volume adapted to the organism's needs. This performance is, essentially, governed by three principal factors: (a) the preload, which may be equated with the ventricular end-diastolic fiber length, (b) the afterload, which is closely related to the intra myocardial systolic tension, and (c) the contractile or inotropic state of the myocardium.[1] The measurement of the stroke volume (i.e., the amount of blood ejected), the ventricular end-diastolic volume and pressure, the systolic ejection time and the Ejection Fraction (EF) permit to evaluate the cardiac performance. However, the value of these measurements is limited in the assessment of the myocardial contractility (which measures the contraction intensity) since they are influenced by alterations in the inotropic state[1] and also greatly affected by alterations in preload and afterload. Thus, the quantification parameters of the contractility should be preload and afterload insensitive.[2]

Heart failure refers specifically to a compromised contractile state of the LV which is accompanied by a forward flow inadequate to accommodate the needs of the peripheral circulation.[3] The overall left ventricular systolic performance is inversely related to the force opposing ventricular fiber shortening (i.e., afterload) and this myocardial property is important in interpreting variables of left ventricular shortening in patients suspected having contractile abnormalities.[4] The reduction in contractile state and the decreased slope of the isovolumetric force-length relationship accounts for the decline in both the extent and rate of fiber shortening for any condition of length or load.[3] This attenuation in shortening implies that the slope of the shortening-length relationship is also reduced.[3] Translated into terms of heart's function as a pump, stroke volume, EF and ejection rate will be reduced. The depression in the maximal force-length values itself represents a reduction in the heart's systolic reserve.[3]

Studies on both animals and humans have suggested that the end-systolic pressure-volume relationship is linear over a physiologic range of loading conditions and is a sensitive indicator of left ventricular contractile function.[5-8] This linear model, originally, proposed by Suga and Sugawa[9,10] is described by the relation

$$P(t) = E(t) \cdot (V(t) - V_o(t))$$

where $P(t)$ is instantaneous pressure inside the LV and $V(t)$ is the Left Ventricular Volume (LVV). $V_o(t)$ is the volume below which the ventricle can no longer generate pressure. Although V_o varies with time from its end-diastolic value (often referred to as "unstressed volume") to its end-systolic value, it varies little near end-systole and can be treated as constant.[8] The changes in V_o may be significantly small or large in diseased hearts. For example, a concentrically hypertrophied ventricle may have a smaller V_o, whereas a chronically volume-overloaded heart may have a V_o considerably larger than normal.[6] The LV is considered as an elastic chamber whose elastance $E(t)$ changes with time. This parameter is an important descriptor of the LV. It increases progressively throughout isovolumetric contraction and left ventricular ejection and then subsequently decreases during isovolumetric relaxation. The maximum elastance that is achieved, E_{max}, represents the slope of the end-systolic pressure/volume line and has been shown to correlate well with measures of contractility.[5] This approach to the analysis of the left ventricular function is hindered by two impediments.[8] First, to measure E_{max} and V_o of the end-systolic pressure-volume relationship, it is necessary to obtain pressure-volume data in a given patient under multiple left ventricular loading conditions without provoking changes in contractility. However, the serial assessment of pressure-volume relationships under changing loading conditions at the present time is difficult with the standard techniques. While the volume data are easily obtained, those of pressure are only obtained invasively. The second impediment is the precise definition of the end-systolic phase. Consequently, the elastance measure is hindered by the need of an invasive technique. It has been shown that there is a positive correlation between E_{max} and EF.[5] The elastance E_{max} is a better index of contractility than the EF although this last one can be achieved more easily.

Global parameters of left ventricular function like EF or volume of LV have been shown to provide important prognostic informations in heart disease[11] and in the evaluation of the cardiac performance. The EF is highly reproducible and provides prognostic informations in patients with coronary artery disease.[12-17] The LVV is one of the most important prognostic factors after acute myocardial infarction.[18,19] An ideal method for the determination of these parameters should be safe, rapid, noninvasive and easily reproducible both at rest and during exercise. Several invasive and noninvasive methods have been reported, none of which can be considered ideal for this purpose.[11] Several techniques are widely used: single and biplane contrast angiography, X-ray computed tomography, M-mode and two-dimensional echocardiography, radionuclide angiography using first-pass studies or gated blood-pool ventriculography and magnetic resonance imaging.[11]

2.2. CARDIAC ANGIOGRAPHY

Since their discovery by Röntgen in 1890, X-ray shadowgraphs have found an increasingly important role in clinical diagnosis. In cardiology, the chest roentgenogram provides a valuable information about the structure and function of the heart and thoracic blood vessels. Imaging of the coronary arteries and the LV chamber by X-ray technique are currently performed in clinical routine. Since, X-rays reflect the variation of electron density in biological tissues, the physiological function is studied by the invasive introduction of a contrast medium. Thus, to visualize the

LV chamber (*Angiography*), the contrast medium is injected through a catheter (*Catheterization*) which passes across the aortic valve into the LV while the heart is exposed to X-radiation. During the cardiac cycle, rapid sequence-radiographs (*Angiogram*) are obtained. The contrast medium filled ventricle is directly measured from the film, during systole and diastole, producing an EF based on changes in LV size. The angiographic procedure is mostly unjustified simply for determination of EF. However, the procedure is often performed along with an angiographic study of the coronary arteries or a cardiac catheterization for study of valvular diseases.[20]

2.2.1. Catheterization

As reported by Cournand,[21] catheterization was first performed (and so named) by Claude Bernard in 1844. The investigation of cardiovascular physiology in animals has led to the development of important techniques and principles including pressure manometry and the application of the Fick principle for measuring cardiac outputs, which are subsequently applied to patients with cardiac disease.[22]

An objective of cardiac catheterization is to assess accurately the forces, and therefore the pressure waves, generated by various cardiac chambers. The information obtained by this technique may be invaluable in the assessment of the LVF. Furthermore, it may yield informations that will be crucial in defining the need for cardiac surgery as well as its timing, risks and anticipated benefit in a given patient.[22]

The catheterization is defined as a combined hemodynamic and angiographic procedure. To perform this procedure, one must take into account the risk of the operation, the consent of the patient and the anticipated value of the information obtained.[22] The procedure is performed using one of the two approaches: catheterization by direct exposure of an artery (brachial vessels ...) or catheterization by percutaneous puncture (including transseptal catheterization).[23] The first approach allows a greater catheter control and a greater selection of catheters. However, this approach can rarely be repeated more than once or twice with safety. In contrast, the second approach, which does not require arteriotomy and arterial repair, can be performed repeatedly in the same patient.[23]

The catheters used are of various diameters, types, lengths and design. Most of them are constructed of Dacron, Polyethylene or Polyurethane. The diameter of a catheter is expressed in French[a] (F) unit. For example, the

---

[a] 1F = 1/3 mm

diameters of the catheters called Gensini, NIH, pigtail, Lehmand and Sones are 7F, 8F, 8F, 8F and 7.5F respectively. The common used catheter for left-heart catheterization is the pigtail catheter, which has multiple side holes and one end hole, and can be used for angiography as well as for pressure measurement. The Sones catheter is designed specifically for coronary arteriography but may also be used for left ventriculography. The Lehman catheter is particulary helpful when dealing with tortuous subclavian artery or stenotic aortic valve. In general, the choice of a catheter size should be suited to the patient's anatomy and the diameters of the catheters vary from 5F to 10F.

For left-heart catheterization, an appropriately selected catheter is inserted into the brachial or femoral artery. This catheter is then advanced into the ascending aorta just above the aortic valve. Once in the ascending aorta, central aortic pressure is measured and recorded simultaneously with arterial monitor pressure. The catheter is then advanced across the aortic valve into the LV. Once the LV has been entered, it is advisable to immediately obtain simultaneous recordings of critical pressures such as left ventricular, peripheral arterial (through the arterial monitor line) pressures etc...

2.2.2. Angiocardiography

Angiocardiography has been used to define the anatomy of the ventricles and related structures and serves as a tool in the study of patients with congenital and valvular heart disease.[24] With increasing frequency, this technique has also been used to evaluate ventricular function, especially to establish prognosis and select patients for coronary artery and valvular surgery.[24] Left ventriculography, which is an essential part of cardiac catheterization, is performed in most patients with known or suspected cardiac disease. It provides important information about the functions of the LV myocardium, the competence of aortic and mitral valves and the presence and location of ventricular aneurysms. Furthermore, it demonstrates anatomical details of the ventricular chamber and associated valves. The left ventriculography procedure is performed from an arterial approach by passing a catheter across the aortic valve into the LV. To achieve adequate opacification of the LV, a relatively large bolus of contrast material is delivered in a relatively short time. The injection rate depends on the size of the LV and the clinical status of the patient.

Digital Substraction Angiography is a method necessitating the injection of smaller quantities of contrast agent and still provides excellent resolution. This method utilizes injection into a peripheral vein, pulmonary artery, or LV.[25] The image acquired before contrast injection (the mask) is substracted from the image obtained after injection. The resulting image represents the structures or regions of interests that one wishes to visualize and quantify.

Quantitative angiocardiography may be carried out using large film or cine techniques (*Cineangiocardiography*), and as biplane or single plane. Cineangiocardiography provides a larger number of sequential observations per unit of time (30 to 60 frames). It allows appreciation of movement and dynamic events through the cardiac cycle and television visualization with filming.[24] The components required in cineangiocardiography include an X-ray generating system, an image intensifier and an image recording system consisting of a video camera, video tape and a cine camera.

2.2.2.1. Generator

The X-ray generator contains a transformer to provide the high voltage necessary to accelerate electrons in the X-ray tube. It also contains another transformer to provide low voltage to heat the tube filament or cathode.

2.2.2.2. X-rays

X-rays are a form of electromagnetic radiation. To produce X-rays, the target of an X-ray tube is bombarded with electrons of high energy. These electrons strike orbital electrons in the inner shells of the target atoms and eject them from their orbits. The vacancy created in an inner orbit is filled by an electron from an outer orbit and this transition is accompanied by emission of an X-ray photon. When the high energy electron does not strike an electron of the target and passes close to the nucleus, it decelerates with change of direction. This deceleration results in X-ray photon emission called "Bremsstrahlung".

2.2.2.3. Image Intensifier

The radiographic image intensifier is a high-gain device for imaging X-ray photons. This device converts the X-ray image into a visible picture of brightness enough to be viewed by a television camera or photographed. The image intensifier and the X-ray tube move in tandem to allow the patient to remain in stationary position and does not have to be subjected to uncomfortable and time consuming repositioning.[26]

2.2.2.4. X-ray Image

In conventional radiography, a patient is placed in front of an X-ray source which transmits radiation through the subject's body. The photons enter the patient where they may be scattered, absorbed or transmitted without interaction. The formed image or "shadow" is a projection of the attenuating properties of all the tissues along the paths of the X-rays. It is a two-dimensional (2D) projection of the three-dimensional (3D) distribution of the X-rays attenuating properties of tissues. Different tissue types in the body exhibit different densities with respect to X-ray radiation. To each tissue density is assigned a physical characteristic value $\mu(x, y, z)$, (x, y, z) being the cartesian coordinates. $\mu(x, y, z)$ is called the linear attenuation coefficient.

Suppose that the incident photons beam is parallel to the z axis and the image is recorded in the $x - y$ plane. Furthermore, we assume that the image may be considered as a distribution of a an absorbed energy. In other words, each photon interacting in the photons detector is locally absorbed. If there are N photons per unit area incident on the patient and $I(x, y)dxdy$ is the energy absorbed in area $dxdy$ of the photons detector, then the image distribution function may be defined as follows:

$$I(x, y) = N\epsilon E \exp\left(-\int \mu(x, y, z)dz\right)(1 + \alpha)$$

where the line integral is over all tissues along the path of the primary photons reaching the point (x, y), E is photons energy and ϵ is energy absorption of the detector. α is the ratio of the scattered to primary radiation that is either measured or calculated.[27] Note that the primary photons recorded form the image (information) and the scattered ones create a background signal which degrades the image contrast.

2.2.3. Projections

Conventional radiography is a limited diagnostic modality in the sense that it produces a 2D projection of a 3D object. However, one may use the adequate projections that provide maximal delineation of the heart structures and minimal overlapping from other structures.

2.2.3.1. Frontal View

In frontal chest X-ray or Postero-Anterior (PA) view, the contour of the normal cardiac structures is predictably outlined against the lung (Figure 5a). The heart image is limited at the left side by the aortic arch, the trunk of the pulmonary artery and the LV, and at the right side by the super vena cava and the right atria. This projection allows to identify hypertrophy of the left cavities.

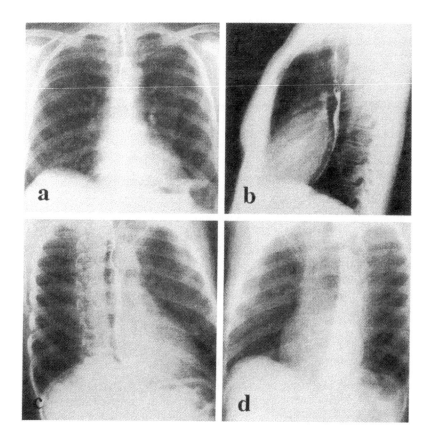

Figure 5. Different views used in conventional cardiology. (a): frontal view, (b): lateral view, (c): right anterior oblique view, (d): left anterior oblique view.

2.2.3.2. Lateral View

In the Lateral (LAT) view, the RV is border-forming in the subxyphoid area and generally extends superiorly about one-third of the distance between the diaphragm and the thoracic apex (Figure 5b). The anterior marging of the pulmonary artery and the ascending aorta lie above the RV.[28] The left atrium forms a shallow convex bulge at the upper aspect of the posterior border of the heart. The normal LV is a long convexity at the posterior-inferior heart border just above the diaphragm.

2.2.3.3. Right Anterior Oblique View

The Right Anterior Oblique (RAO) is performed with the patient in 45° right anterior projection in relation to the film (Figure 5c). In this view, there is an elongation of the ventricles so that the long axis of the ventricles are in view and the atrioventricular groove is in profile.[28] The advantage of the RAO projection is to eliminate overlapping of the ventricle and spine and puts the mitral ring in profile. This view is helpful to the angiographer in determining the presence or absence of mitral and tricuspid regurgitation and stenosis.

2.2.3.4. Left Anterior Oblique View

The Left Anterior Oblique (LAO) view is performed with the patient in the 60° oblique (Figure 5d). This view obviates overlapping of the aortic valve and spine and allows visualisation of the ventricular septum. This projection is a useful angiographic view to diagnose the presence of LV enlargement.

In some cases, it may be advisable to perform ventriculography in two separate projections. For example, both RAO and LAO (biplane angiography) may be required in the evaluation of suspected ventricular aneurysm.[24]

2.2.4. Assessment of Ventricular Function

Assessment of ventricular function, performance and contractility is important in the evaluation of many patients with known or suspected heart disease. Thus, measures such as preload, ventricular volume, dimensions, intracardiac pressures, wall stress and fractional shortening are necessary.

2.2.4.1. Left Ventricular Volume

Measurement of ventricular volume is a standard technique to assess LV function. One of the most widely used approach for calculating LV volume is the area-length method introduced by Dodge et al.[29] They have suggested that the ellipsoid is the most representative figure for the LV and that the dimensions of this figure can be determined from angiograms taken in perpendicular planes (Figure 6). In this method, LAT and Antero-Posterior (AP) projections (Figure 7) of the LV outline are used to compute the volume, using the formula:

$$V = \frac{\pi}{6} \cdot L \cdot D_{AP} \cdot D_{LAT}$$

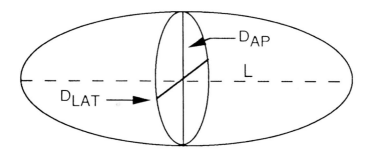

Figure 6. Ellipsoid model used to calculate left ventricular volume.

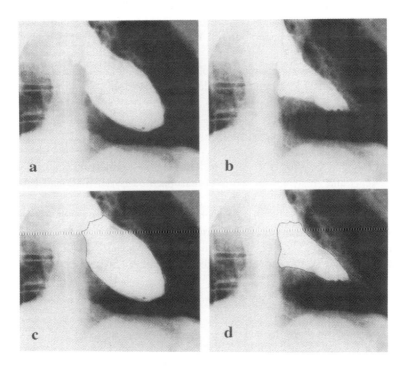

Figure 7. The anteroposterior (a) and lateral (b) biplane angiocardiograms. The left ventricular cavity is outlined in black on the anteroposterior (c) and lateral (d) views.

L is the longest length in centimeters in AP or LAT projections of the ventricular chamber (i.e., from the apex to the root of the aortic valve). D_{AP} and D_{LAT} are the diameters (minors axes) of the ventricle calculated from the AP and LAT projections. The L, D_{AP}, D_{LAT} are magnified by virtue of divergent X-ray beams, and therefore must be corrected before substitution into the volume relation. The diameter D from each plane (i.e., LAT or AP) is calculated as follows:

$$D = \frac{4A}{\pi L}$$

A is the area of the opacified LV cavity and can be conveniently determined by a hand or electronic planimeter and X-Y plotter. The calculation of A is made for images exposed in both AP and LAT projections.

The LV contours obtained from angiographic image[30–32] by manual tracing may be derived by automatic techniques. Manual tracing is tedious and time consuming and dependent on the technical skill of the operator. Thus, some automatic methods of varying difficulty and complexity have been proposed for computer generation of LV contours from digital angiographic images.[33–38]

In practice, biplane angiograms are obtained in the 30° RAO and 60° LAO projections. Thus, LV volume is calculated using the following formula:[39]

$$V = \frac{8}{3\pi} \cdot \frac{A_{RAO} - A_{LAO}}{L_{min}}$$

where L_{min} is the shorter L value in RAO or LAO projection (Figure 8), and A_{RAO} and A_{LAO} are the areas of the opacified LV in RAO and LAO respectively.

The LV volume is estimated for each image of the cardiac cycle. ED and ES are selected as the largest and smallest volumes respectively. The LV Stroke Volume (SV) is defined as the difference between ED Volume (EDV) and ES Volume (ESV) and the EF as the ratio between SV and EDV:

$$EF = SV/EDV$$

2.2.4.2. The Ventricular Pressure-Volume Relation

Additional information can be obtained concerning the functional characteristics of the LV by relating LV volume to LV pressure (Figure 9)

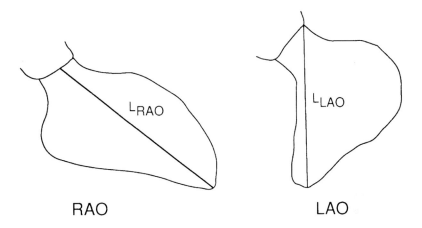

RAO   LAO

Figure 8. Diastolic left ventricular silhouettes of right anterior and left anterior obliques cineangiograms.

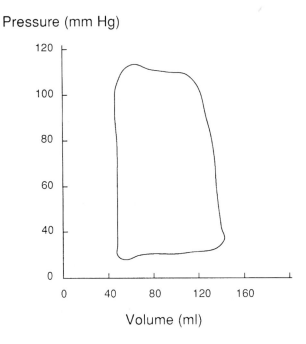

Figure 9. Simultaneous pressure and volume measurements are related to construct a pressure-volume diagram.

recorded during or immediately prior to angiocardiography.[40] Characteristic changes in the LV pressure-volume loops occur in various disease states. The pressure-volume diagram reflects the phases of the cardiac cycle beginning at ED and followed by isovolumic contraction, systolic emptying, isovolumic relaxation and diastolic filling. The area subtended by the systolic portion of the curve provides a measure of stroke work performed by the LV during systole, whereas the area subtended by the diastolic limb provides a measure of diastolic work performed on the LV by distending it during diastole.[39]

2.2.5. Ventricular Wall Motion

LV contractile abnormalities can be an important manifestation of coronary artery disease. These wall motion changes may represent ischemia or infarction of myocardium.[41] The quantification of the extent of regional wall motion abnormalities may help in determining the myocardial effects of coronary disease. Contrast angiography and other imaging techniques permit study of ventricular wall motion. In current clinical practice, wall motion can be appreciated by visual inspection of cineventriculograms. The poor reproducibility of such an evaluation had led to the development of quantitative methods that measure the extent of wall motion at different points around the endocardial contour (Figure 10).[42–45]

2.2.6. Conclusion

Angiocardiography is a standard method for evaluating LV function. This method is a routine part of the cardiac catheterization. It is an accepted technique for measuring ventricular cavity volumes and intraventricular pressures. However, this procedure is invasive and not free of discomfort or risk and most importantly, it is usually not suitable for repeated applications at close intervals in the same patient. Furthermore, angiographic contrast medium may affect the LVF. The immediate hemodynamic effects include increases in cardiac output, LV ED pressure and pulmonary capillary wedge pressure.

2.3. COMPUTED TOMOGRAPHY

A problem with conventional X-radiography is the loss of depth information. The 3D anatomical structure is collapsed or projected into a 2D film. With the introduction of Computed Tomographic (CT) X-ray technique,[46] the interest of X-ray methods has immediately been increased. In X-ray CT, a planar slice

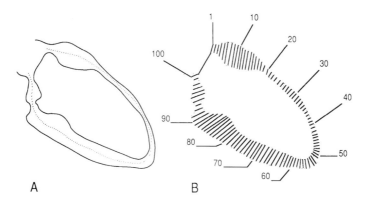

Figure 10. Centerline technique of regional wall motion analysis. (A) End-diastolic and end-systolic left ventricular endocardial outlines and centerline generated automatically midway between the two contours. (B) Motion is measured along 100°chords constructed perpendicular to the centerline.

of the body is defined and X-rays passed through it only in directions that are contained within and are parallel to the plane of the slice. The resulting image shows the human anatomy in section with a good spatial resolution and density (linear attenuation) distribution of better than 1%.[47] The CT scan consists of a series of 2D axial slices of an organ (e.g., heart) which may be stacked to form a 3D representation. The acquisition of this 3D representation is done noninvasively. CT imaging modality is based on the same physical principle than that of the conventional radiography.

In a common X-ray CT configuration, there are an X-ray source and an array of X-ray detectors. These two elements are connected in a fixed collinear arrangement forming a gantry. The source-detector combination measures parallel projection one sample at a time by stepping linearly across the patient. After each projection, the gantry rotates to a new position for the next projection. The gantry rotation allows the acquisition of line integrals of tissue density along multiple paths. In general, the gantry is rotated a full 180° around the patient with a sufficient number of density measurements collected to reconstruct the anatomical cross-section. The most well-known reconstruction method in CT is the standard Filtered BackProjection (FBP). This method performs image reconstruction from X-ray (line integral) projection data. Once each slice is reconstructed, using FBP algorithm, the resulting slices are stacked to form the 3D representation. For example, usually 10 to 12 tomographic slices are needed to encompass the heart entirely.

2.3.1. CT Image Reconstruction

The CT image reconstruction consists of determining the density distribution $g(x, y)$ in the $x - y$ plane, given some subset of projections $p(\theta, t)$ in the plane. $p(\theta, t)$ is the value of the integral along the line passing through $(t \cos \theta, t \sin \theta)$ in the direction normal to θ and is given by:

$$p(\theta, t) = \int_{-\infty}^{+\infty} \int_{-\infty}^{+\infty} g(x, y)\delta(x \cos \theta + y \sin \theta - t)dxdy$$

where δ is the Dirac function. With a sufficient number of projections collected between zero and π, the function, $g(x, y)$, can be correctly reconstructed by backprojecting filtered versions of the projections.[48] The filtered projections are given by:

$$Q(\theta, t) = \int_{-\infty}^{+\infty} P(\theta, f) \mid f \mid e^{j2\pi ft}df$$

where $P(\theta, f)$ is the Fourier transform of $p(\theta, t)$ given by

$$P(\theta, f) = \int_{-\infty}^{+\infty} p(\theta, t)e^{-j2\pi ft}dt$$

The operation of backprojection for reconstructing slice data set, $g(x, y)$, is described by

$$g(x, y) = \int_{0}^{\pi} Q(\theta, x \cos \theta + y \sin \theta)d\theta$$

An example of a heart cross-section reconstructed slice is shown in Figure 11. To each element (pixel) in the slice matrix is assigned a CT number which is a measure of the density, with respect to water, of the tissues located in this point.

Thus, with the FBP reconstructed images, the volume of the organ scanned can be formed. This CT volumetric data sets can be obtained at high-speed with an X-ray CT scanner known as Dynamic Spatial Reconstructor (DSR).[49] The DSR provides dynamic synchronous volume 3D CT images, every 1/60 seconds. This system consists of 14 X-ray sources mounted at 12 degree intervals around a circular gantry. A cone beam of X-rays is transmitted from each source to 2D detectors. In its highest temporal resolution mode, the DSR generates 14 projections through the cross-section of interest in 1/100 second, and repeated recording of new sets of 14 projections every 1/60 second.[50]

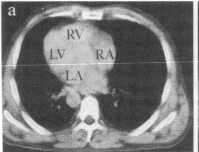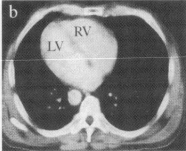

Figure 11. Heart cross-sections reconstructed by FBP algorithm. X-ray CT scan at the level of the sinus of Valsalva (a). X-ray CT scan where the septum is well visible between the two ventricles (b).

2.3.2. Cine-CT

CT scanning of the heart requires modification of the standard CT technique used for investigating anatomy characterized by little motion. Indeed, CT does not provide adequate information about moving structures due to mechanical limitations and time acquisition required. The shortest time needed to collect data transmitted from many angles of single rotating X-ray source is of the order of 1–2 seconds. During this lenght of time, the heart beats at least once and the CT reconstructions are therefore blurred.[50] One approach to overcome the difficulties posed by the heart motion is the use of the "gated scanning technique".[51] The ECG gating methodologic strategy has enhanced the application of CT to cardiac investigation. This method involves recording the subject's ECG during the length of time, generally spanning many heart cycles, for which projection data are recorded. Subsequent to scanning, those projections, recorded during different heart cycles but at the same instant of the cycle as determined from the ECG, are grouped together to reconstruct an image of the heart corresponding to the selected timepoint in the cardiac cycle.[50] The fundamental assumption underlying this technique is that the 3D changes in location, size, shape and density of the cardiac structures are repeated in an identical, reproducible manner for many heart cycles. This assumption is of questionable validity in even healthy hearts, and is almost certainly invalid in the study of abnormal cardiac dynamics, which involve considerable beat-to-beat variability.[50] Another approach to this problem is the ultrafast (Cine) CT scanner.[52] This system permits to obtain scans at exposure times of 50 msec or less and can generate CT scans at multiple anatomical levels. The ultrafast scanning speed (50 msec/slice) has made CT a viable noninvasive modality to image cardiac structures. The Cine-CT scanner employs a scanning focused X-ray beam, which provides complete cardiac imaging in real time without the need for ECG gating. This CT system is not limited by the inertia associated with moving mechanical parts. It uses a focused electron beam that is successively swept across four cadmium tungstate target arcs.[53] Each of the four targets generates a fan beam of photons that pass from beneath the patient to a bank of photon detectors arranged in a semicircle above the patient.

2.3.3. Evaluation of Cardiac Function

Measurement of LV EF is a widely utilized parameter of LV function that reflects the hemodynamics and prognosis of a variety of cardiovascular diseases. For this reason, there is much interest to determine LV EF accurately and provide the clinician with this valuable information. The accurate determination of EF necessitates precise measurements of ED and ES volumes. In angiocardiography, measurement of theses volumes is adversely affected by lack of sharpness of ventricular borders and varying spatial orientation of the LV. Furthermore, the use of single geometric reference (ellipsoid) to fill all possible ventricular shapes may not be appropriate.[52] Cine-CT has the potential ability to precisely measure LV volume with cross-sectional imaging of consecutive tomographic slices of the ventricle irrespective of geometric shape. The measure of ED and ES volumes results in good estimation of stroke volume and EF. Cine-CT can be applied for simultaneous quantification of the RV and LV volumes. It can demonstrate LV segmental dysfunction such as reduced wall thickening and wall motion. Futhermore, Cine-CT is a useful noninvasive method for the visualization of cardiovascular anatomy in patients with congenital heart disease and can provide assessment of their cardiovascular function.[53]

Prior to the investigation, intravenous injection of iodinated contrast medium is used to delineate the blood pool on CT scans. The contrast medium can be given as intravenous bolus injection. A series of short-axis (tomograms) from apex to the base, to encompass the heart, are acquired during multiple phases of the cardiac cycle. The acquisition performed with an interscan delay of order of 8 msec. Thus, real-time sequential imaging is accomplished within a single heart beat and the acquired images are then displayed in a closed-loop cine format (Cine-CT display).

Endocardial edges of the LV can be determined visually based on the different CT numbers between the LV cavity and myocardium. These edges can be outlined manually in diastole (largest area) (Figure 12a) and systole

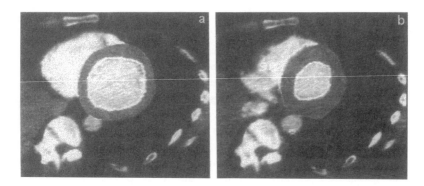

Figure 12. CT short axis tomograms. Manual tracing of the endocardial edge in end-diastolic (a) and end-systolic (b) frames.

(smallest area) (Figure 12b). Since manual tracing is time consuming and puts strict constraints on the amount of data that can be processed, many automatic and semi-automatic methods have been proposed.[36,54–58] The tomographic measurements of ED and ES volumes at each level are added by the use of modified Simpson's formula. EF is then determined by calculating the ratio between the stroke volume and ED volume. It has been demonstrated that LV volume, EF and stroke volume acquired by Cine-CT are of high accuracy and close reproducibility among observers and among studies on different occasions in the same patient.[52]

2.4. ECHOCARDIOGRAPHY

Echocardiography is a highly attractive clinical tool in cardiological diagnosis. The cross-sectional imaging of the heart has been standardized and physiological data such as LVV or EF have been extracted from such images.[59] This noninvasive technique permits to observe both cardiac structures and motion. The echocardiography is the most readily available imaging method for bedside risk after acute myocardial infarction.[60–62] Because it delivers no ionizing radiation, assessment echocardiography is particularly valuable for the study of pregnant females, children and females of child bearing age. Besides the absence of tissue damage, the other advantages of the echocardiography are low cost, minimal discomfort and real time processing.

2.4.1. Principle

Unlike the other imaging techniques, ultrasound is a *contact* procedure. Before examination, a thin film of an acoustical gel is applied to the patient skin. The hand-held transducer passes over the skin gliding along the gel. The echocardiography depends on penetration of the body by high-frequency sound, emanating from the transducer and bouncing off internal structures. The returning sound beam ("echo") is perceived by the transducer and built into an image.[63] The same transducer is used for both transmission and detection. Ultrasound source/detector configurations can consist of a single transducer or an array of transducers. These array configurations provide a larger receptor aperture and subsequently improved image reconstruction. The spatial information of this image, due to the physical nature of the imaging system, is basically represented by speckles[b] or blotches of relative gray-level intensity. Boundary speckles represent existing physical borders and can vary in size and in the distance between them.

Because air does not transmit diagnostic ultrasound, the heart cannot be imaged through most of the chest wall. However, by careful transducer angulation, the sound beam can be directed through the anterior mediastinum and bounced back ("echoed") from the endocardial surfaces, pericardium and cardiac valves.[63]

Most diagnostic applications of ultrasound are based on the pulse-echo method. Pulse-echo data may be displayed in many different ways. The display methods are:

2.4.2. A-mode

A-mode (Amplitude-mode) is based on the reflexion of the ultrasound pulses displayed on the screen by amplitude modulation which is used for one-dimensional measurements of distances. The information is shown on the screen in the form of echo amplitudes plotted versus depth.

2.4.3. B-mode

B-mode (Brightness-mode) is based on the composition of reflected pulses displayed on the screen by brightness modulation, which is used for two-dimensional scans. The information is shown on the screen in the form of brightness versus depth.

---

[b] "Speckle" is the term used for an analogous phenomenon observed is coherent laser light.

2.4.4. M-mode

In M-mode (Motion-mode), an echo range displacement (depth) versus time type of display is added to the basic B-mode for the purpose of recording and measuring dynamic structures. This mode possesses high ultrasonic sampling rates in the time domain that are directed forward and back along a single path. This representation mode, time-histogram record, permits recording of an amplitude and the rate of motion objects with great accuracy. Consequently, it can record the most rapid events, such as valve opening or closing.[64] The simultaneous display of a series of sequential cardiac cycles allows a rapid visual and mental integration of data that speeds interpretation. The M-mode Echocardiography (ME) is the original technique for the cardiac examination. It is useful for evaluating left ventricular performance and measuring LVV in patients without regional myocardial dysfunction.[65] The ME technique is particularly suited for analysis of motion, dimension and thickness of various structures, such as septum, posterior wall, cardiac valves and dimensions of the aorta, Left Atrium (LA) and LV. It is helpful in aortic stenosis and insufficiency, cardiomyopathies, pulmonary stenosis and insufficiency and right ventricular volume overload.[66]

In performing a sweeping from the apex to the heart basis, the cardiac structures are continuously recorded and analysed according to the three classical lines: transventricular, transmitral and transaortic (Figure 13).

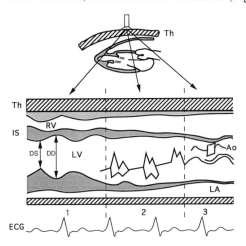

Figure 13. Diagrammatic presentation of an M-mode echocardiogram as the transducer is directed from the apex to the base of the heart (Th: Thoracic anterior wall, RV: Right Ventricle, LV: Left Ventricle, IS: Intraventricular Septum, LA; Left Atrium, Ao: Aorta, DD: Diameter of the left ventricle in Diastole, DS: Diameter of the left ventricle in Systole).

2.4.5. Derived ME Measurements

A number of derived parameters are calculated from the ME left ventricular measurements:

2.4.5.1. *Percent Fractional Shortening (PFS%)*

The PFS of the minor axis of the LV is determined as follows:[67,68]

$$\text{PFS\%} = \frac{DD - DS}{DD} \times 100\%$$

where DD and DS are the left ventricular internal dimensions at ED and at ES. This parameter, PFS%, is easy to calculate and useful to evaluate the global left ventricular function. It varies in normal cases from 28% to 45%.

2.4.5.2. *Left Ventricular Volume*

LVV is measured according to the American Society of Echocardiography convention:[69]

$$\text{LVV} = \frac{3.14 \times DD^3}{3}$$

Using ME, a considerable amount of information concerning cardiac anatomy, chamber diameter, wall thickness and even estimation of the EF can be obtained. However, because of its unidimensional limitation and the loss of spatial resolution, it is difficult to assess motion in the lateral walls of the ventricle (i.e., motion perpendicular to the ultrasonic beam), chamber shape and to obtain reliable volume calculation and EF. An ultrasonic method that may circumvent these limitations is the two-dimensional echocardiography which provides additional cross-sectional information.

2.4.6. Two-Dimensional Echocardiography

Two-Dimensional Echocardiography (2DE) is a valuable tool for quantitative analysis of cardiac function. It derives indexes of LVF by measuring LVV and EF.[70,71] The determination of the LVV and the related hemodynamic parameters play an important part in estimating prognosis in chronic valvular and myocardial disease. 2DE has overcome some of the methodological problems of ME. The base of the heart as well as the whole LV can be imaged. This technique features tomographic images of the heart in real time, allows beat-to-beat evaluation of chamber geometry, internal structures and

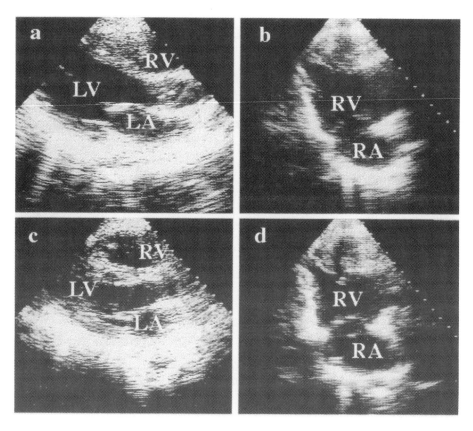

Figure 14. 2DE images. Parasternal long axis images: diastolic image (a) and systolic image (b). 2DE of the Right Atrium (RA) and Right Ventricular (RV) inflow tract: diastolic image (c) and systolic image (d).

motions of the wall. Because 2DE image anatomically represents the heart (Figure 14), potentially more useful information may be derived from 2DE than ME.

2.4.7. Principle

The LV is imaged in four planes using a transducer mechanically (or electronically) swept at a given frequency through an arc of adjustable width.[65] By moving the ultrasonic beam very rapidly, a sector scan of the moving structure would be obtained with correct spatial orientation

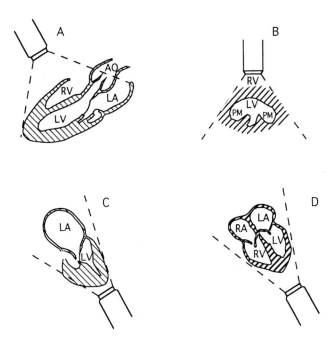

Figure 15. Diagrams demonstrating the four standard tomographic planes obtained from four different transducer positions: long-axis view (A), short axis view (B), axial view (C) and four-chamber view (D).

and cardiac shape and lateral motion could be depicted. Depending on the measurement sought, four standardized tomographic planes are obtained:[65]

The long-axis view is obtained from the third, fourth or fifth intercostal space along the left sternal border, with the sector plane parallel to the long axis of LV (Figure 15A). *The short-axis* view is obtained from the same position as the long-axis view by rotating the transducer 90° so that the sector plane is perpendicular to the long-axis and the left ventricular cavity appears circular (Figure 15B). *The axial* view is obtained with the transducer at the apex of the LV and the sector plane directed to transect the true anterior and posterior walls of the LV and the LA (Figure 15C). *The four-chambers* view is obtained from the same position by rotating the transducer 90°.[65] In this view, the posterolateral and septal walls of the LV and the four cardiac chambers can be imaged (Figure 15D).

Computer processing of the acquired 2DE images allows estimation of LVVs and derived functions such as EF as well as motion analysis. Images are selected at ES and ED phases. ES is defined as the frame at which the reference ECG reaches the end of the T wave or the frame just before the opening of the mitral valve.[72] ED is defined as the frame at which the reference ECG reached the peak of the R wave or the frame just before the closing of the mitral valve.

2.4.7.1. *Left Ventricular Volume*

LVV may be computed from the dimensions and area measurements obtained from the paired apical views (that is, four-chamber and two-chamber), which may be considered orthogonal for the purposes of quantitation.[73] Two methods may be used.

The biplane method

This method is also called modified Simpson's rule. The calculation of the volume results from summation of areas from diameters $e_1(i)$ and $e_2(i)$ of n cylinders or discs of equal height. This method treats the ventricle as a stack of slices which are apportioned by dividing left ventricular longest into n equal sections (Figure 16).

$$V = \frac{\pi}{4} \sum_{i=1}^{n} e_1(i) \cdot e_2(i) \cdot \frac{L}{n}$$

This method is less sensitive to geometric distorsions. One approach to compute the $e_1 2(i)$ or $e_3(i)$ values is to correctly outline the LV contours (Figure 17) and then to generate the n cords. For automatic contours detection of the LV, several approaches have been proposed.[63,74–79]

The single plane method

This method is applicable when only one apical view is of adequate quality. The volume is calculated assuming a prolate ellipsoid geometry.

$$V = 0.85 \frac{A^2}{L}$$

where L and A are the endocardial length and the area of the left ventricular cavity respectively. The LVV at ED (EDV) and at ES (ESV) are estimated and the EF calculated using the following formula:

$$EF = \frac{EDV - ESV}{EDV} \times 100\%$$

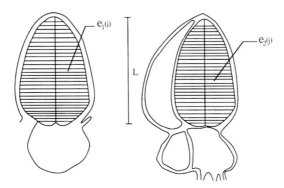

Figure 16. Biplane method of discs (modified Simpson's rule) based on nearly orthogonal planes from apical two- and four-chamber views.

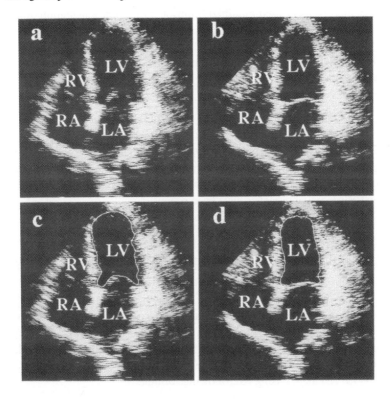

Figure 17. 2DE four-chamber: diastole (a) and systole (b). Manual tracing of the left ventricle in diastole (c) and systole (d).

2.4.7.2. The Fractional Area Change

The rapid computer data acquisition facilitates frame by frame analysis of changes in 2DE cross-sectional area throughout the cardiac cycle. Derivatives of such curves during systole and diastole may serve as indicators of LV ejection and filling rates respectively.[80] A systolic Fractional Area (FA) change is readily calculated from these curves and serves as a parameter of regional function.

$$FA = \frac{EDA - ESA}{EDA} \times 100\%$$

where EDA and ESA are the 2DE cross-sectional areas in diastole and systole respectively.

2.5. RADIONUCLIDE VENTRICULOGRAPHY

One of the earliest use of the radioactive material for diagnostic tests on patients was reported by Blumgart and Yens.[81] They have measured the arm-to-arm circulation time using a small quantity of radium-C ($\simeq$ 100 MBq). The beta emission was detected with a Wilson cloud chamber.[82] One of the advantages of the use of radionuclide in medicine is the large signal (the emitted radiation) obtained from a relatively small mass of radionuclide employed for a given study.[83] Nuclear medicine takes advantage of this physical characteristic by using various radioisotope-tapped compounds (radiopharmaceuticals) to trace various functions of the body. Thus, cardiac performance can be assessed with radionuclide technique. Radionuclide ventriculography provides a noninvasive way to evaluate ventricular function both visually and quantitatively. Since its introduction in 1971,[84] electrocardiographically gated cardiac blood pool imaging has gained widespread clinical acceptance for the noninvasive assessment of the LVF.

2.5.1. Instrumentation

The acquisition and processing of radioisotope imaging studies in cardiovascular nuclear medicine are performed with a scintillation camera interfaced to a computer. The first electronic gamma camera with multiple PhotoMultiplier (PMT) tubes was reported in 1958 by Anger.[85] The Anger camera or gamma camera is the instrument of choice for radioisotope imaging. The visual display of radioactivity is a result of photon passing through three principal camera units including a collimator, a large sodium iodide crystal of varying thickness (from 6 mm to 9 mm) and an array of 37 to 91 PMT tubes.[86]

2.5.1.1. Collimator

The collimator restricts the field of view of the detector to the small volume of material immediately beneath it. Since gamma rays are emitted isotropically, there is no inherent relationship between the position at which a gamma ray interacts with the scintillation crystal and its emission point in the patient. The collimator approximates the origin of the photon emission within the patient to an analogous location within the crystal.

2.5.1.2. Detector

Materials that emit visible light when energy is absorbed from ionising radiation can be used to count and image radioisotopes. Light emission by most inorganic scintillators is proportional to energy deposit in the material. Hence, it is possible to detect photons using a scintillation counter and to determine the energy of the photon detected.[87] NaI(Tl) crystal is used as a scintillation detector. Most modern detector systems consist of stacked circular detector arrays. The detector crystal produces an electrical pulse when it is stricken by a gamma photon. Indeed, when a gamma-ray photon enters the crystal, a fast electron is formed due to either photoelectric effect or Compton scattering with the crystal's ions. This radiation is sensed by a PMT tube and converted to an electrical pulse.

2.5.2. Radiopharmaceuticals

The radiopharmaceuticals used for radionuclide imaging are compounds which will be metabolised or incorporated into the human tissue to be studied. The distribution of these agents, within the body, is determined by the route of administration and by such factors as blood flow, blood volume and a variety of metabolic processes. The choice of radionuclide will be made on the basis of suitable emission and half-life, while the compound will be chosen for appropriate biochemical, physiological or pharmacological properties.[82] The half-life of the radionuclide is fundamental in determining the radiation dose to administer to the patient. The most widely used generator-produced radionuclide in nuclear medicine is ^{99m}Tc. Its physical half-life of 6 hours and gamma energy of 140 keV are ideally suited for current gamma cameras. Radionuclide ventriculography may be performed by first-pass or equilibrium techniques. Radiopharmaceutical requirements for the first kind of studies are

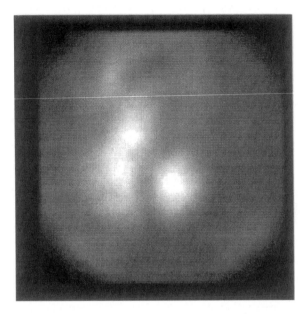

Figure 18. Left anterior oblique projection: end-diastolic frame.

a high photon flux at low delivered radiation dose. Clinically, ^{99m}Tc-labeled pharmaceuticals are most often used for this purpose. Since the agents cross the lungs after intravenous injection, they permit measurements of the LVF.[17] For equilibrium measurements, the radiopharmaceuticals should have an unchanging concentration in the blood pool during the interval of measurement. Two ^{99m}Tc-labeled agents, red blood cells and albumin, meet this criteria.

2.5.3. Views

For visual and quantitative analysis of cardiac performance, multiple views may be used. These include the standard anterior and Left Anterior Oblique (LAO) as well as the left lateral and left posterior oblique views. The LAO view (Figure 18) provides data for the quantitative assessment of LVF. In this view, the two ventricles are spatially well separated. The degree of left anterior obliquity must be individualized based upon specific patient anatomy and cardiac orientation within the thorax. The LAO view also provides qualitative information concerning contraction of the septal, inferor, apical and lateral walls.[86] The anterior view provides data concerning regional motion of the anterior and apical segments. The left lateral or left posterior oblique views provide optimal qualitative information concerning contraction of the inferior wall and postero basal segment.[86]

2.5.4. Assessment of Cardiac Performance

Radionuclide Ventriculography (RNV) techniques are used for the noninvasive evaluation of cardiac function. Cardiac function measurements can be obtained by two RNV techniques. The first involves analysis of the first transit of radionuclide bolus through the central circulation (first-pass technique). The second, involving analysis following equilibrium intravascular labeling allows repeated imaging over several hours (equilibrium technique).[86] These two techniques are reliable to evaluate global and regional parameters of ventricular function.

2.5.4.1. First-Pass Technique

With the first-pass technique, 10–20 mCi of ^{99m}Tc pertechnetate are injected intravenously as a compact bolus. Subsequently, the radioactivity is measured during the first-pass of the tracer through the central circulation as it moves into the RA, RV, pulmonary artery, lungs, LA and LV.[87] The radionuclide data may be recorded as a sequence of images (ungated) or in synchrony with the patient's ECG (gated). The gated first-pass technique uses R-wave of the ECG as time marker to separate different beats and provides the temporal and anatomical separation of the RV and LV. The data are recorded for 30–60 seconds and afterwards 5 to 10 cardiac cycles are summarized to form an average cycle. By generation of a time activity curve, one can determine LVEF and RVEF based on changes in radioactivity over time. The first-pass approach is well suited for left to right shunt detection and for qualitative assessment of regional wall motion abnormalities and can be performed both at rest and during exercise.[87] The efficacy and reliability of this method depends on obtaining sufficiently high count rates to ensure statistical reliability.

2.5.4.2. Equilibrium Radionuclide Technique

After injection (5 to 10 minutes) of an equilibrium radiopharmaceutical (20–25 mCi), data are recorded in synchrony with the R-wave of the patient's ECG. Using the multiple gated acquisition approach, every cardiac cycle is divided into 16–32 frames. Data are accumulated until radioactivity count density is sufficient for statistically meaningful analysis. From these data, a time-activity curve can be generated over LV and LVEF estimated.[88] The equilibrium technique can be applied both at rest and during exercise. Imaging at rest is performed at, at least, two positions (anterior and optimal – best separation – LAO). The combination of high count density and multiple views (anterior, LAO and left posterior oblique) enhances the sensitivity of equilibrium images for the detection of wall motion abnormalities.

2.5.5. Radionuclide Acquisition

Radionuclide data are acquired and stored in either list or frame mode. In list mode, information is arranged as serial spatial and temporal data and can later be reordered into dynamic data files (frame mode). In the frame mode, which is employed most frequently, the R-R interval of ECG is divided into 20 to 50 msec portions, depending upon the patient's intrinsic heart rate and the conditions of the study (rest or exercise).[86] For example, in the first-pass study, one can store the spatial information (x, y) for each detected event and timing parameter (t). This temporal information (t) can be used in subsequent reordering of the data into a series of time-dependent frames.[83]

Imaging is carried out using a 20% window centered on the 140 keV photopeak of ^{99m}Tc and a beat rejection window of $\pm 10\%$ using dynamic arrhythmia filtration.[89] For assessment of the LVF, the imaging is performed in LAO projection providing best separation of the two ventricles. The scintigraphic images are stored in $64 \times 64 \times 16$ bits format. The acquired images are degraded by multiple factors such as the collimating system, the statistical fluctuations and the photon counting process. Noise in scintigraphic images is most evident at high spatial frequencies. Thus, a filter to attenuate high frequencies while sparing low frequencies is necessary. One of the most frequently used smoothing filter in nuclear medicine is a nine-point array of weighting factors representing a pseudo-Gaussian filter shape:[82,90]

$$\begin{pmatrix} 1 & 2 & 1 \\ 2 & 4 & 2 \\ 1 & 2 & 1 \end{pmatrix}$$

2.5.6. Background Activity

Radioactivity is present within the entire intravascular structures. Major contributions of this background comes from lungs, left atrium and, to a lesser extent, chest wall.[86] Thus, it is necessary to correct for the contribution of activity in adjacent intravascular structures to the overall measured LV radioactivity. In the LAO projection, the LA is posterior to the LV and it will have its background contribution attenuated substantially by the more anterior left ventricular blood pool. Consequently, left atrial activity does not have a major impact on LV measurements.[86] In clinical routine, a background region is drawn manually and can also be obtained automatically.[90]

2.5.7. Count-Based Method

The most widely used method to estimate ventricular volume is the count-based method.[91] The radioactivity recorded from a chamber, at equilibrium, is proportional to the volume of the chamber (when neglecting radiation tissue absorption). The stroke volume counts are directly related to the stroke volume measured invasively. A correction for attenuation of blood pool activity by overlying chest wall is necessary. The count-based method is independent of geometric considerations and allows the use of automatic edge detection methods to compute the EF from the LAO images on equilibrium studies. Recently, a new count-based approach to calculating volume that does not involve attenuation correction has been described. This method may simplify substantially current volumetric analysis.[92]

2.5.8. Data Processing

Gated cardiac blood pool imaging is a well-established technique for the assessment of LVF. The most widely used parameter to characterize quantitatively the LV performance is the global EF. It is highly reproducible and provides prognostic information in patients with coronary artery disease.[16] The values of EF obtained by either first-pass or equilibrium techniques are comparable.[17] The EF is best calculated using the count-based technique. To compute the EF, a gated sequence of 16 images is collected at each cycle over several hundred cycles and filtered.[90] A region of interest is assigned over the LV using either manual, threshold, second derivative or phase analysis algorithm to define the contours of the LV in each frame. In the semi-automatic method, a rectangular window surrounding the LV in the ED frame is manually positioned and its size adjusted by a user.[90] Once the window is well positioned (Figure 19), a zero crossing, a second derivative edge tracking algorithm is used beginning with the present image until the end of the sequence. In searching for the edge of the LV, the algorithm starts in the center of the window until a matrix point is reached that satisfies one of the two conditions. An edge is detected if a point is a zero crossing or if a point has a count value less than an user selected threshold value (55% of the maximum count in the window). The edge search is limited to the window.

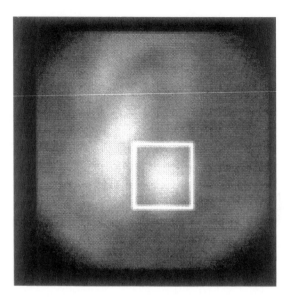

Figure 19. A window surrounding the left ventricle in the end-diastolic frame.

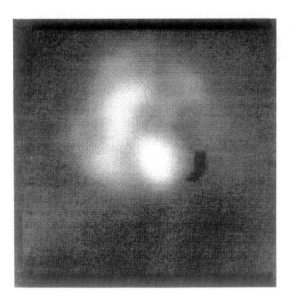

Figure 20. Automatic placement of the region of interest for background noise subtraction.

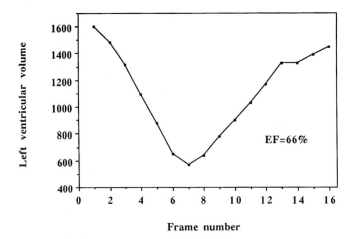

Figure 21. Graph of the left ventricular function.

Since a proportion of the total counts measured in the LV region of interest arise from outside the LV, a background region is generated lateral and inferior to the LV[90] (Figure 20). The counts in the background region are computed and normalized to the LV area. From LV region of interest, a background corrected LV time-activity curve is obtained (Figure 21). The systolic frame is located by finding the minimum of this curve. The EF is calculated by dividing the stroke counts by the background corrected ED counts. As alternative to semi-automatic method, several automatic methods have been proposed.[90,93-97] In [90], the Fuzzy C-Means (FCM) clustering algorithm and a Fourier Analysis are used for automated detection of the LV contours. The computation begins by finding the phase image (Figure 22). The FCM is first applied to this image to generate a number of clusters which correspond to the heart substructures (LV,...). Second, the ventricles cluster (LV and RV) is isolated and the intensities of its points are replaced by the corresponding ones from the original ED frame (Figure 23). Finally, a reduced image representing the ventricular region is obtained and an additional clustering is performed to find automatically the LV edges (Figure 24).

2.5.9. Systolic and Diastolic Ventricular Function Parameters

Four parameters can be derived from left ventricular time-activity curve (V) to characterize diastolic ventricular function. To obtain these parameters,

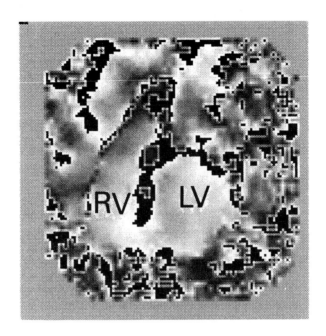

Figure 22. Phase image: Result of the Fourier analysis performed on the sequence of 16 frames.

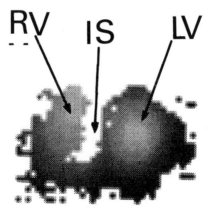

Figure 23. Reduced image representing the ventricular region (LV: Left Ventricle, RV: Right Ventricle, IS: Intraventricular Septum).

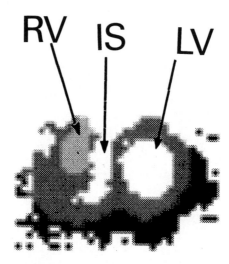

Figure 24. Result of the final fuzzy clustering applied to the reduced image (LV: Left Ventricle, RV: Right Ventricle, IS: Intraventricular Septum).

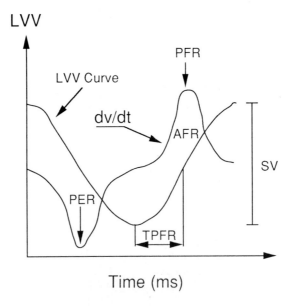

Figure 25. Plot of the left ventricular volume (V) versus time and the rate of change of volume (dV/dt) versus time obtained by radionuclide ventriculography (PER: Peak Ejection Rate, PFR: Peak Filling Rate, SV: Stroke Volume, TPER: Time to Peak Ejection Rate, TPFR: Time to Peak Filling Rate).

the derivative of the function, V, is generated. This curve (Figure 25) identifies the areas of the peak ejection and the peak filling and the times of their occurrence.[98] The four parameters are the Peak Ejection Rate (PER), the Peak Filling Rate (PFR), the Time-to-Peak Ejection Rate (TPER) and the Time-to-Peak Filling Rate (TPFR):

$$PER = \max\left(\frac{-dV}{dt}\right)$$

$$PFR = \max\left(\frac{dV}{dt}\right)$$

the PFR is the most widely applied parameter of diastolic function and is often viewed as an index of LV compliance. It reflects global ventricular diastolic properties. TPER is the difference between the time to ED and the time of PER. TPFR is the difference between the time to ES and the time of PFR. The TPFR parameter is viewed as index of LV relaxation.

2.5.10. Regional Wall Motion

LV performance can be characterized qualitatively for wall motion abnormality by visual assessment of an endless cinematic loop of the cardiac cycle. From inspection of the cinematic display regional wall motion is assessed. This inspection permits, subjectively, grading of regional wall motion, for instance on a four-point scale with 1 being normal, 2 hypokinetic, 3 akinetic and 4 dyskinetic, based on comparisons of ED to ES outlines. A total score for the LV is then derived.

2.5.11. Fourier Analysis

The complex information represented by the sequence of 16 frames per cycle can be reduced into two images, namely phase and amplitude images, representing both anatomy and physiology. The stroke volume image provides useful data but does not take full advantage of the cyclic nature of the gated blood pool scan. Phase and amplitude images are generated by Fourier analysis, a more elaborate technique, used for cardiac contraction kinetic.[90] The analysis is done on each time-activity curve. Since the primary assumption of Fourier analysis is that the data is periodic, the transition between the first and the last frame of the study must be smooth. Each pixel in the frame sequence is considered to be curved in time. The time-activity curve represents a relatively simple repeating function. The pixel time activity is approximated by its first harmonic.[90]

Let $Sora(i, j, k)$ be the value of the pixel (i, j) of the k-th frame. Two images, I_{cos} and I_{sin} are calculated:

$$I_{cos}(i, j) = \sum_{k=1}^{16} \cos\left[\frac{2\pi}{16}(k-1)\right] \cdot Sora(i, j, k)$$

$$I_{sin}(i, j) = \sum_{k=1}^{16} \sin\left[\frac{2\pi}{16}(k-1)\right] \cdot Sora(i, j, k)$$

The phase and amplitude images are given, respectively, by:

$$I_{phase}(i, j) = \arctan\left[\frac{-I_{sin}(i, j)}{I_{cos}(i, j)}\right]$$

$$I_{ampl}(i, j) = \left[I_{cos}^2(i, j) + I_{sin}^2(i, j)\right]^{\frac{1}{2}}$$

The phase image reflects the timing of regional ejection and enables us to isolate cardiac chambers and their contraction pattern free of background (Figure 22). By definition, the phase values of the ventricular (RV and LV) contractions are distributed around 0 degree. Since the atria contract before the ventricle, atria pixels are out of phase (approximately 180 degrees) with ventricles. The amplitude image is qualitatively similar to the stroke volume where the atria can be detected. Fourier analysis will never replace the subjective evaluation of the cinematically displayed data by an experienced observer but yields additional quantification which has important clinical applications.

2.5.12. Gated Single Photon Emission Computed Tomography

Planar radionuclide ventriculography shares the same difficulty as all imaging modalities using projection images. Important structures in such images may be hidden or masked by other objects in front of or behind them. Thus, true ventricular volumes cannot be performed. A new approach to measure true three-dimensional ventricular volume by Gated Single Photon Emission Computed Tomography (GSPECT) of the intracardiac blood pool is proposed.[99,100] Furthermore, GSPECT allows visualization of the four-dimensional distribution (three cartesian coordinates and time) of the radionuclide in the heart. GSPECT is a natural extension of planar gated blood pool scanning and rotating camera SPECT technology.

After red blood cell pool labeling with an adequate quantity of ^{99m}Tc pertechnetate using an *in vivo* or *in vitro* technique,[101] the patient is placed supine on the imaging table and heart rate is sampled to measure the mean R-R interval for selecting ES and detecting the presence of arrhythmia.[102] The study is acquired in 64×64 image matrix during $180°$ rotation from $45°$ right anterior oblique to $45°$ degrees left posterior oblique. Each projection image set is acquired at a temporal resolution of 16 frames equally distributed over the entire cardiac cycle. Gated tomography projection image sets are reconstructed into transverse sections using FBP algorithm as in X-ray CT. A ramp Butterworth filter can be used. The tomographic sections are orthogonal to the long axis of the LV. In each tomographic section, the LV is isolated.[103] By summing the areas of LV sections, both ED and ES volumes are derived. The GSPECT method has obviously an advantage over planar imaging as it makes no assumptions about the shape of the ventricle. The preliminary results reported by Faber *et al.*[104] show that motion quantification from GSPECT images can be performed. A clinical experience has demonstrated the superiority of GSPECT over planar blood pool images for precise definition of subtle functional abnormalities.[100] In addition to single photon, gated blood pool tomography can also be performed with positron emitting tracers and data can be recorded with gated positron tomographs.[105] The use of positron technique improves image resolution and allows better quantitation of cardiac volumes.

2.6. MAGNETIC RESONANCE IMAGING

It is well established that the cardiac catheterization technique is the "*gold standard*" for the assessment of the EF and the LVV. However, this technique is invasive and requires the use of contrast medium. The radionuclide ventriculography is non-invasive but requires radiopharmaceutical preparations. Echocardiography is employed more frequently with less risk and discomfort but the imaging quality is, to a great extent, dependent on obtaining an adequate cardiac window. Magnetic Resonance (MR) imaging provides a non-invasive method and requires no conventional contrast medium for determining the LVV and the EF. MR imaging gives an excellent contrast between the flowing blood and myocardium. It can be used to obtain images of the heart at any angle and provides accurate LV long and short axis sections. This imaging technique is of high spatial resolution to depict correctly the cardiac anatomy. Furthermore, it provides the temporal resolution needed to obtain precise evaluations of cardiovascular function.[106]

2.6.1. Principle

MR imaging is applied to atomic nuclei with an odd number of protons or neutrons or both. Only nuclei with these characteristics can be made to resonate and give rise to MR signal. The simplest nucleus is that of the Hydrogen (^{1}H) atom, which consists of one particle only, the proton. ^{1}H is the most common element found in biological tissue, concentrated in tissue water. It has a high abundance and has a high sensitivity to its MR signal. That is why the ^{1}H MR imaging is largely used.

When imaging the human body, the spinning protons in an organ (heart...) align either parallel or antiparallel with externally imposed static magnetic field, B_0. The protons align with the field and simultaneously experience a torque due to B_0. As a result, they precess about B_0 axis at a rate given by the Larmor equation:

$$\omega = \gamma B_0$$

where γ is the gyromagnetic ratio. This parameter expresses the nucleus sensitivity to MR signal. This sensitivity increases proportionally with the signal frequency. For example, ^{1}H has the largest γ and therefore has the largest MR signal sensitivity. ω is the frequency of the Electromagnetic (EM) energy required to cause a transition between the two different spin states. The Larmor equation defines the resonance frequency at which the nuclei absorb energy. The protons pointing in the parallel direction are at a slightly lower energy than those pointing in the antiparallel direction. The energy difference, ΔE, between states is given by:

$$\Delta E = \gamma \hbar B_0$$

where $\hbar$ is the Planck's constant (h) divided by 2π. ΔE value is the energy absorbed or emitted in the form of the EM radiation. A short time after the application of B_0, the number of protons pointing in the parallel direction is very slightly higher than the number of those pointing in antiparallel direction and the sample (tissue...) is said to be magnetized. This excess parallel state population is represented by the net magnetization vector, $\overrightarrow{M}$. In clinical imaging with MR, the energy required to stimulate or excite a low-energy parallel proton to a higher antiparallel proton is the EM waves in the Radio-Frequency (RF) scale.[107] Thus, if in B_0 field, RF waves of right frequency are passed through the volume, some of the parallel protons will absorb energy and will be stimulated or excited to higher energy in the antiparallel direction. At some time later, the exact RF frequency absorbed will be emitted as EM energy of the same frequency as the RF source. The protons continue to absorb-emit (i.e., to resonate), as long as the radio waves have the correct resonant frequency.[107]

Prior imaging, $\overrightarrow{M}$ is in its equilibrium position, aligned along the z axis of the gantry and there is no detectable MR signal. Note that B_0 is by convention aligned along the z axis of a three-dimensional coordinate system. The MR receiver coils are oriented such that only the component of $\overrightarrow{M}$ in the transverse (x, y) plane induces a measurable signal. Components of $\overrightarrow{M}$ in the transverse direction are referred to as transverse magnetization and the components along the z axis as longitudinal magnetization. During the imaging process, RF pulses modify $\overrightarrow{M}$. This interaction results in the emission of RF energy which is detected in the receiver coils. The emitted RF energy is referred to as the MR signal.

To create an MR image, the anatomic region (heart...) under study is placed in three powerful magnetic fileds: a static uniform field, B_0, a pulse or RF field, B_1, and a static non-uniform (gradient) field. These fields excite tissue in such a way that it emits very weak RF radiation. Transverse magnetization is created by B_1, applied in the transverse plane. The flip angle denotes the displacement over which $\overrightarrow{M}$ is rotated from equilibrium after the application of the RF signal. This angle, θ, is given by the relationship:

$$\theta = \gamma B_1 t_p$$

where t_p is the time duration of the RF pulse. Different combinations of RF pulses and timing relationships constitute a MR pulse sequence. Within every pulse sequence, there is a specific time interval, T_E (Time Echo), during which MR data is acquired. Via proper selection of T_E it is possible to obtain good contrast between various tissue types whether normal or pathological. Image is produced by applying the sets of RF pulses many times over several minutes. The time between application of sets of RF pulses is called the Repetition Time (T_R). The emitted RF radiation is detected, computer-stored and constructed into an image. The image can be formed in any plane through the volume of interest: transverse, longitudinal, frontal and oblique. The appearance of any given tissue on the image (i.e., black, gray or white) can be drastically changed by varying the pattern of RF pulses. Furthermore, the RF pulses are brief and can be synchronized with the ECG for cardiac motion studies via "gating".

Useful informations from tissues can be extracted using pulse sequences. Varying tissue-related factors influence the emitted MR signal. The most important of these are the relaxation times. The relaxation is the time process by which the spins respond to the disrupting effects of both their environment and external RF pulses. There are two relaxation times denoted by T_1 (spin-lattice) and T_2 (spin-spin). Through proper RF stimulation, it is possible to acquire information regarding one of the two tissue characteristics, T_1 and T_2.[108] MR images, created from sequences emphasizing T_1 (T_2) information, are called T_1 (T_2) weighted images.

T_2-weighted images can be obtained by the Spin Echo (SE) technique. Images are produced by sampling signal after an initial 90° RF pulse, followed by one or more 180° pulses. The 180° pulse refocuses spins and thereby enhances the signal from them. The signal is sampled some time after the 180° pulse. Another method by which images are acquired more rapidly than with SE imaging by reducing T_R value is the Gradient-Echo (GE) sequence. This technique uses a short T_R and a flip angle less than 90°.[109] This reduction is achieved by switching off the read gradient to focus the signal rather than by a time-consuming refocusing of the RF pulse. In SE imaging sequence, blood appears black on images; therfore, internal structures of the heart can be visualized within the signal void of the cardiac chambers. Using the GE technique, the blood pool appears white and has substantially higher signal than the myocardium, again providing good edge definition of the endocardial margin.

The common concept to the methods used to obtain T_1-weighted images is to observe the longitudinal magnetization at various times in its recovery process due to T_1 effects. Among the methods used are Saturation Recovery (SR) and Inversion Recovery (IR). The efficient form of SR sequence is repeated SE sequence with "spoiler" gradient pulses applied between repetitions. These gradients disperse the transverse magnetization from the preceding 90°–180° pulses. The gradient amplitudes are randomized to avoid formation of extra echoes. In SR, a first 180° pulse inverts the longitudinal magnetization which then recovers for a time T_1 until it is observed with a 90°–180° SE combination.

2.6.2. Cardiac Triggering

Acquisition of MR signals of the thorax without gating results in poor cardiac images owing to two factors. The first is the loss of the signal from moving structures while the second is the variable position of the cardiac structure relative to imaging pixels when data are acquired indiscriminately throughout the cardiac cycle.[109] Cardiac triggering is used to minimize the effects of the heart's motion during data acquisition. ECG leads are attached to the patient lying inside the magnet. To achieve an ECG signal that will reliably trigger the MR acquisition, the electrodes are optimally positioned. Each profile is started at a specific time, governed by trigger pulses derived from the R tops of the ECG signal. The rapid rise in the ECG signal, indicating the beginning of the R wave, generates a trigger pulse. The measurements are

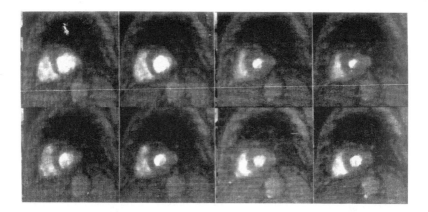

Figure 26. Cine-MR images acquired in the short axis plane at different positions of the heart (only 8 positions are represented).

started immediately after reception of the R wave pulse or after some variable time delay to coincide with a later phase of the heart cycle.

2.6.3. Imaging Methods

2.6.3.1. Multiple Phase Scanning

The R-R interval is used to acquire a number of heart phase images (Figure 26). This is achieved by detecting the first R peak and after a short trigger delay, a number of excitations will occur before the next R peak is detected. Each of these excitations will be performed at the same point in time after the R peak in the successive R to R intervals until all matrix data are acquired to construct a number of heart phase images. Multi Phase (MP) can be combined with single slice or multiple slices in Fast Field Echo (FFE) and for SE, either Single Slice Multi Phase (SSMP) or Cycled Multi Slice Multi Phase (CMSMP). The MP scanning allows the display of the cardiac data as a movie and to be used in quantitative regional wall motion analysis. The SE Multi Slice method can be used as a survey and for an overview of morphology and visualization of aneurysms and stenosis. SE-SSMP method is used for analysis of diastolic and systolic phases of the cardiac cycle. The FFE-SSMP and the FFE-MSMP methods are used to study the ventricular function.

2.6.3.2. Tissue Tagging

The advance in high speed imaging allows to obtain cross-sectional images in short periods of time. Thus, it is possible to generate MR images rapidly enough to study the motion of tissue between consecutive frames.[110] The tissue contours are identified using edges detection algorithms and the motion of these contours are tracked. The motion seen is just that of the inner and outer surfaces of the tissue. The motion of the tissue between the surfaces is not known. This is a limitation of the tomographic methods which do not permit to track the same point in the myocardium throughout the cardiac cycle.[111] This limitation is the result of the complex motions (translation, rotation, twist, tilt, shear, shortening) of the heart and the absence of landmarks in the myocardium.[112] Identifiable and trackable landmarks are needed within the tissue, just as the contours, are for the outside of the tissue. Recently, a method has been developed for magnetically "tagging" different regions of the heart wall so that their motion may be followed with MR imaging.[111] MR tags are produced by a RF pulse, referred to as the tagging pulse, applied in conjunction with pulsed magnetic field gradients. The heart is subjected to the additional RF pulse just before the slice and/or phase excitation RF pulse. The tagging RF pulse can be applied in a grid or line pattern. This pattern, when viewed over successive heart phases, will move with the heart and demonstrate normal versus abnormal heart wall motion (Figure 27). The tagging technique, introduced by Zerhouni et al.,[111] is a two-stage process. In the first stage, a set of non-invasive tags is placed in the tissue through a perturbation of the equilibrium magnetization. In the second stage, the position of the tags and the surrounding tissue is imaged as a function of time.[113] The deformation observed in the tags directly reflects the deformation of the underlying tissue that has occurred in the time elapsed between placing the marker and imaging the myocardium.[113] Furthermore, the cardiac tagging technique is being developed to map the three-dimensional deformation of large segments of the myocardium over the entire LV during contraction in the normal and ischemic heart.[112]

2.6.3.3. Cine MR Imaging

This can be accomplished by ECG referencing of fast imaging sequences. Cine MR imaging is a pulse sequence with partial flip angles and gradient-refocused echoes.[113] This approach can produce approximately 30 images (20 to 30 msec duration) during the cardiac cycle (Figure 26). The images are laced together in a cinematic display so that a wall motion of the ventricles, valve motion, and blood flow patterns in the heart and great vessels can be visualized.[109] Volume of three-dimensional data acquisition is also achieved

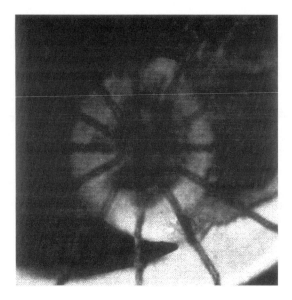

Figure 27.   Tagged left ventricle image at end-diastole.

with an ECG-gated sequence. With this technique, images of any desired plane can be reconstructed later, and all reconstructed planes are in the same phase of the cardiac cycle (in contrast to the multislice technique).[109]

2.6.4.   Cardiac Exams Views

In order to perform adequate cardiac exams, views must be planed along the true axis of the heart. For a given clinical investigation, an appropriate view is chosen and angulation adjusted to suit the individual patient. Among the views currently used in cardiac exams are:

2.6.4.1.   Short Axis

The SA LV view is often used to access wall motion in the ventricle because the wall and the septum can be seen in profile. In this view, the LV and RV are spatially well separated (Figure 26). This view is accomplished with single or double angulation through the heart. The angulation degree depends on the anatomical configuration and pathology. SA view is used in multiple slice/multiple phase sequences. The acquired data are used to estimate

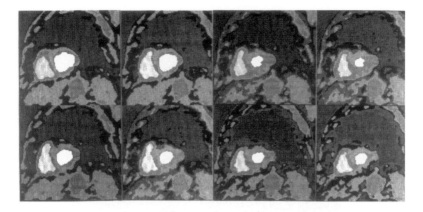

Figure 28. Result of fuzzy segmentation of the 8 cine-MR images.

the LVV and the SV. SA images are considered optimal for quantitating ventricular dimensions.

2.6.4.2. Long Axis

The long axis view is used to see connections between AT and ventricles or ventricles and vessels, and to investigate the valve function between these structures. Like the SA view, the long axis is performed with either single or double angulations. This view is used to determine the area length EF.

2.6.5. A Cardiac Analysis Method

We have, for instance, evaluated LV function using measurements obtained from Cine-MR imaging. This technique employed a flip angle of $30°$ and gradient refocused echoes with an echo (T_E) of 123 msec. The T_R is equal to 21 msec. ECG-gated multislice and multiphase technique is used. The field of view and the slice thickness are of 350 mm and 10 mm respectively. The acquisition matrix is 128×256 interpolated to 256×256 for display. The imaging is performed with 0.5T Philips scanner. SA images are obtained at 10 different positions (slices) and 20 time intervals (phases) during the cardiac cycle. Figure 26 shows 8 images among 10 corresponding to 8 phases of the middle plane of the cardiac cavity. These images are filtered using median filter. An automated method, based on the FCM algorithm[114] to delineate the LV region, is used[115] (Figure 28). Interesting methods to perform this

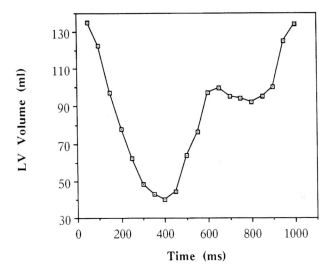

Figure 29. Plot of the left ventricular function.

image processing have been proposed.[116–119] For each phase of the cardiac cycle, the different cross-sectional area of the LV are calculated. Volumes are estimated for each phase by adding the areas multiplied by slice thickness and the LV function curve calculated (Figure 29). The ES volume corresponds to the minimum of this curve. The LV parameters of the study are the following:

$$EDV = 135 \text{ ml}$$
$$ESV = 40 \text{ ml}$$
$$SV = 95 \text{ ml}$$
$$EF = 70\%$$

2.7. CONCLUSIONS

In this chapter, we have briefly presented the techniques used to assess the LVF. The assessment can be performed with echocardiography, radionuclide ventriculography, angiocardiography, Cine-CT and MR imaging. The use of any cardiac imaging technique should be based on appreciation of the types of information it provides. Angiocardiography is the standard for chamber volume against which the other imaging techniques are judged.

Because of its portability and safety, echocardiography is used as the initial tool to assess LVF. It is a technique of choice to estimate LVF in the intensive care unit or emergency department. With the advent of transoesophageal echocardiography, cardiac chambers can be accurately assessed. Radionuclide technique, even not extremely precise for calculation of LVV, is well accepted for determination of LV systolic and diastolic performance. Indeed, this technique does not require geometric assumption like Cine-CT, echocardiography and MR imaging. It also does not require detailed definition of endocardial and epicardial LV contours. In the case where precise determination of LVV is needed, the use of Cine-CT and MR imaging methods are necessary. These two techniques are slightly more accurate and produce more detailed images of cardiac anatomy than echocardiography and radionuclide ventriculography. However, Cine-CT and MR imaging have, at present, the disadvantage of being expensive.

Remark

I apologize to all whose work I have inadvertently omitted in this review.

2.8. ACKNOWLEDGEMENTS

I gratefully acknowledge Pr. R. Itti, chief of Nuclear Medicine Center (Lyon), for his interest in this work and for his helpful suggestions. I wish to express my sincere thanks to Pr. J.J. Mallet, responsible of GRISN (EA 640) research group (Lyon), for the use of computer/display facilities to produce data figures shown in this chapter. I would like to thank Dr. J. Champier, research scientist at Claude Bernard University (Lyon), for his careful reading and critical review of the manuscript. Thanks are also due to Dr. J.C. Bordet, research scientist at Pasteur Institute (Lyon), for data acquisitions and to Dr. S. Durbin, Dr. M. Crozet and Dr. Z. Hamici for their encouragements.

2.9. REFERENCES

1. Mason, D.T., E. Braunwald, J.W. Covell, E.H. Sonnenblick and J. Ross, 1971, *Circulation*, **44**, 47–58.
2. Comet, M. and J. Machecourt, 1988, *J. Med. Nucl. Biophys.*, **12**, 17–28.
3. Weber, K.T. and J.S. Janicki, 1979, *Am. Heart. J.*, **98**, 371–384.
4. Lang, R.M., K.M. Borow, A. Neumann and D. Janzen, 1986, *Circulation*, **74**, 1114–1123.
5. McKay, R.G., J.M. Aroesty, G.V. Heller, H.D. Royal, S.E. Warren and W. Grossman, 1986, *Circulation*, **74**, 97–104.
6. Sagawa, K., 1978, *Circ. Res.*, **43**, 678–686.
7. Mehmel, H.C., B. Stockins, K. Ruffmann, K.V. Olshausen, G. Scheller and W. Kübler, 1981, *Circulation*, **63**, 1216–1222.

8. Sagawa, K., 1981, *Circulation*, **63**, 1223–1227.
9. Suga, H. and K. Sagawa, 1973, *Circ. Res.*, **32**, 314–322.
10. Suga, H. and K. Sagawa, 1974, *Circ. Res.*, **35**, 117–126.
11. Al-Khawaja, I.M., A. Lahiri and E.B. Raftery, 1988, *Nucl. Med. Commun.*, **9**, 495–504.
12. Burggraf, G.W. and J.O. Parker, 1975, *Circulation*, **51**, 146–156.
13. Proudfit, W.L., A.V.G. Bruschke and F.M. Sones, 1978, *Prog. Cardiovasc. Dis.*, **21**, 53–78.
14. Harris, P.J., F.E. Harrell, K.L. Lee, V.S. Behar and R.A. Rosati, 1979, *Circulation*, **60**, 1259–1269.
15. Hammermeister, K.E., T.A. DeRouen and H.T. Dodge, 1982, *Circulation*, **65**, 53–59.
16. Jones, R.H., R.D. Floyd, E.H. Austin and D.C. Sabiston, 1983, *Ann. Surg.*, **197**, 1983, 743–753.
17. Rocco, T.P., V. Dilsizian, A.J. Fischman and H.W. Strauss, 1989, *J. Nucl. Med.*, **30**, 1149–1165.
18. White, H.D., R.M. Norris, M.A. Brown, P.W.T. Brandt, R.M.I. Whittock and C.J. Wild, 1987, *Circulation*, **76**, 44–51.
19. Jeremy, R.W., R.A. Hackworthy, G. Bautovich, B.F. Hutton and P.J. Harris, 1987, *J. Am. Coll. Cardiol.*, **9**, 989–995.
20. Grossman, Z.D., D.A. Ellis and S.C. Brigham, 1983, *The Clinician's Guide to Diagnostic Imaging* (Raven Press, New York).
21. Cournand, A., 1975, *Acta. Med. Scand. Suppl.*, **579**, 1–32.
22. Grossman, W., 1992, In *Heart Disease. A Textbook of Cardiovascular Medicine* (E. Braunwald ed.) (W.B. Saunders Company, Philadelphia) 4th ed., Chap. 7, pp. 180–203.
23. Grossman, W., 1980, *Cardiac Catheterization and Angiography* (Lea and Febiger, Philadelphia), 2nd ed., Chap. 1, pp. 3–10.
24. Hood, W.P., C.E. Rackley and W. Grossman, 1980, In *Cardiac Catheterization and Angiography* (W. Grossman ed.) (Lea and Febiger, Philadelphia), 2nd ed., Chap. 14, pp. 170–184.
25. Nissen, S.E., D. Booth, J.Waters, T. Fassas and A.N. DeMaria, 1983, *Am. J. Cardiol.*, **52**, 1293–1298.
26. Levin, D. and L. Dunham, 1980, In *Cardiac Catheterization and Angiography* (W. Grossman ed.) (Lea and Febiger, Philadelphia), 2nd ed., Chap. 2, pp. 11–24.
27. Dance, D.R., 1988, In *The Physics of Medical Imaging* (S. Weeb ed.) (Adam Hilger, Bristol and Philadelphia), Chap. 2, pp. 20–71.
28. Steiner, R.M. and D.C. Levin, 1992, *Heart Disease. A Textbook of Cardiovascular Medicine* (E. Braunwald ed.) (W.B. Saunders Company, Philadelphia), 4th ed., Chap. 8, pp. 204–234.
29. Dodge, H.T., H. Sandler, D.W. Ballew and J.D. Lord, 1960, *Am. Heart J.*, **60**, 762–776.
30. Heintzen, P.H., V. Malerczyk, J. Pilarczyk and K.W. Scheel, 1971, *Comput. Biomed. Res.*, **4**, 474–485.
31. Alderman, E.I., H. Sandler, J.Z. Brooker, W.J. Saunders, C. Simpson and D.C. Harrison, 1973, *Circulation*, **47**, 309–316.
32. Cole, J.S., D.D. Brown and D.H. Glaeser, 1974, *Comput. Biomed. Res.*, **7**, 575–589.
33. Chow, C.K. and T. Kaneko, 1972, *Comput. Biomed. Res.*, **5**, 388–410.
34. Pope, D.L., D.L. Parker, D.E. Gustafson and P.D. Clayton, 1984, *Comput. Cardiol.*, 71–75.
35. Lilly, C.K., M. LeFree, E. Anselmo, S. Tehrani, J. Jenkins and P.D. Bourdillon, 1985, *Comput. Cardiol.*, 257–260.
36. Lilly, P., J. Jenkins and P. Bourdillon, 1989, *IEEE. Trans. Med. Imaging*, **8**, 173–185.
37. DeFigueiredo, M.T. and J.M.N. Leitao, 1992, *IEEE. Trans. Med. Imaging*, **11**, 416–429.
38. Demi, M., 1994, *Comput. Biomed. Res.*, **28**, 157–177.
39. Brunwald, E., 1992, *Heart Disease. A Textbook of Cardiovascular Medicine* (W.B. Saunders Company, Philadelphia), 4th ed. Chap. 15, pp. 419–443.
40. Dodge, H.T., H. Sandler, W.A. Baxley and R.R. Hawley, 1966, *Am. J. Cardiol.*, **18**, 10–24.
41. Gelberg, H.J., B.H. Brundace, S. Glantz and W.W. Parmley, 1979, *Circulation*, **59**, 991–100.

42. Sheehan, F.H., E.L. Bolson, H.T. Dodge, D.G. Mathey, J. Schofer and H.W. Woo, 1986, *Circulation*, **74**, 293–305.
43. Von Land, C.D., S.R. Rao and J.H.C. Reiber, 1991, *Proc. Computers in Cardiology, IEEE Comp. Soc.*, 483–486.
44. Coppini, G., M. Demi, R. Calmai and G. Valli, 1992, *J. Biomed. Eng.*, **14**, 321–328.
45. Baroni, M., 1994, *Comput. Methods Programs Biomed.*, **42**, 33–38.
46. Hounsfield, G.N., 1973, *Br. J. Radiol.*, **46**, 1016–1022.
47. Swindell, W. and S. Webb, 1988, In *The Physics of Medical Imaging* (S. Webb. ed.) (Adam Hilger, Bristol and Philadelphia), Chap. 4, pp. 98–127.
48. Crawford, C.R. and A.C. Kak, 1979, *Applied Optics*, **18**, 3704–3711.
49. Robb, R.A., E.A. Hoffman, L.J. Sinak, L.D. Harris and E.L. Ritman, 1983, *Proc. IEEE*, **71**, 308–319.
50. Garden, K.L. and R.A. Robb, 1986, *IEEE Trans. Med. Imaging*, **5**, 233–239.
51. Sagel, S.S., E.S. Weiss, R.G. Gillard, G.N. Hounsfield, R.G.T. Jost, R.J. Stanley and M.M. Ter-Pogossian, 1977, *Invest. Radiol.*, **12**, 563–566.
52. Reiter, S.J., J.A. Rumberger, A.J. Feiring, W. Stanford and M.L. Marcus, 1986, *Circulation*, **74**, 890–900.
53. Higgins, C.B., 1992, In *Heart Disease. A Textbook of Cardiovascular Medicine* (E. Braunwald ed.) (W.B. Saunders Company, Philadelphia), 4th ed. Chap. 11, pp. 312–341.
54. Higgins, W.E., N. Chung and E.L. Ritman, 1989, *SPIE Visual Communications and Image Processing IV*, **1199**, 932–943.
55. Higgins, W.E., N. Chung and E.L. Ritman, 1990, *IEEE Trans. Med. Imaging*, **9**, 384–395.
56. Taratorin, A.M. and S. Sideman, 1993, *IEEE Trans. Med. Imaging*, **12**, 512–533.
57. Chen, C.W., J. Luo, K.J. Parker and T.S. Huang, 1995, *Comput. Med. Imaging Graph.*, **19**, 85–100.
58. Tu, H.K., A. Mathemy, D.B. Goldgof and H. Bunke, 1995, *Comput. Med. Imaging Graph.*, **19**, 27–46.
59. Clas, W., R. Brennecke, R. Zotz, R. Erbel, D. Jung and J. Meyer, 1987, *Int. J. Cardiac Imag.*, **2**, 111–116.
60. Heger, J.J., A.E. Weyman, L.S. Wann, J.C. Dillon and H. Feigenbaum, 1979, *Circulation*, **60**, 351–538.
61. Nishimura, R.A., A.J. Tagjik, C. Shub, F.A. Miller, D.M. Illstrup and C.E. Harrison, 1984, *J. Am. Coll. Cardiol.*, **60**, 1080–1087.
62. Berning, J. and F. Steensgaard-Hansen, 1990, *Am. J. Cardiol.*, **65**, 567–576.
63. Friedland, N. and N. Adam, 1989, *IEEE. Trans. Med. Imaging*, **8**, 344–353.
64. Kisslo, J., 1979, *Circulation*, **60**, 734–736.
65. Carr, K.W., R.L. Engler, J.R. Forsythe, A.D. Johnson and B. Gosink, 1979, *Circulation*, **59**, 1196–1205.
66. Grube, E., M. Zywietz, B. Backs and C. Reifahrt, 1981, *Medical Ultrasonic Images* (C.R. Hill and A. Kratochwil eds.) (Excerpta Medica, Amsterdam-Oxford-Princeton) Chap. 16, pp. 134–141.
67. Quinones, M.A., E. Pickering and J.K. Alexander, 1978, *Chest*, **74**, 59–65.
68. Gardin, J.M., N.D. Wong, W. Bommer, H.S. Klopfenstein, V.E. Smith, B. Tabatznik, D. Siscovik, S. Lobodzinski, H. Anton-Culver and T.A. Manolio, 1992, *J. Am. Soc. Echocardiogr.*, **5**, 63–72.
69. Devereux, R.B. and N. Reichek, 1977, *Circulation*, **55**, 613–618.
70. Helak, J.W. and N. Reichek, *Circulation*, **63**, 1981, 1398–1407.
71. Kuecherer, H.F., L.L. Kee, R.N. Gunnard, M.D. Cheittin and N.B. Schiller, 1991, *J. Am. Soc. Echocardiogr.*, **4**, 203–214.
72. Huang, Z.H., W.Y. Long, G.Y. Xie, O.L. Wan and A.N. DeMaria, 1992, *Am. Heart. J.*, **123**, 395–402.
73. Shah, P.M., M. Crawford, A. DeMaria, R. Devereux, H. Feigenbaum, H. Gutgesell, N. Reickek, D. Sahn, I. Schnittger, N.H. Silverman and A.J. Tajik, 1989, *J. Am. Soc. Echocardiogr.*, **2**, 358–367.

74. Adam, D., O. Harenveni and S. Sideman, 1987, *IEEE Trans. Med. Imaging*, **6**, 266–271.
75. Chu, C.H., E.J. Delp and A.J. Buda, 1988, *IEEE Trans. Med. Imaging*, **7**, 81–90.
76. Klingler, Jr. J.W., C.L. Vanghan, T.D. Fraker and L.T. Andrews, 1988, *IEEE Trans. Biomed. Eng.*, **35**, 925–935.
77. Freng, J., W.C. Lin and C.T. Chen, 1991, *IEEE Trans. Med. Imaging*, **10**, 187–199.
78. Han, C.Y., K.N. Lin, W.G. Wee, R.M. Mintz and D.T. Porembka, 1991, *IEEE Trans. Med. Imaging*, **10**, 602–610.
79. Coppini, G., R. Poli and G. Valli, 1995, *IEEE Trans. Med. Imaging*, **14**, 301–317.
80. Garcia, E., P. Gueret, M. Bennett, E. Corday, W. Zwehl, S. Meerbaum, S. Corday, H.J.C. Swan and D. Berman, 1981, *Am. Heart J.*, **101**, 783–792.
81. Blumgart, H.L. and O.C. Yens, 1927, *J. Clin. Invest.*, **4**, 1–13.
82. Sharp, P.F., P.P. Dendy and W.I. Keyes, 1985, *Radionuclide Imaging Techniques* (Academic Press, INC. London).
83. Ott, R.J., M.A. Flower, J.W. Babich and P.K. Marsden, 1988, In *The Physics of Medical Imaging* (S. Weeb ed.) (Adam Hilger, Bristol and Philadelphia), Chap. 6, pp. 142–318.
84. Strauss, H.W., B.L. Zaret, P.J. Hurley, J.K. Natarajan and B. Pitt, 1971, *Am. J. Cardiol.*, **28**, 575–580.
85. Anger, H.O., 1958, *Rev. Sci. Instrum.*, **29**, 27–33.
86. Zaret, B.L., F.J. Th. Wackers and R. Soufer, 1992, In *Heart Disease. A Textbook of Cardiovascular Medicine* (E. Braunwald ed.) (W.B. Saunders Company, Philadelphia) 4th ed. Chap. 10, pp. 276–311.
87. Felipe, R.F., H. Prpic, J.W. Arndt, E.E. Van der Wall and E.K.J. Pauwels, 1991, *Eur. J. Radiol.*, **12**, 20–29.
88. Wackers, F.J., H.J. Berger, D.E. Johnstone, L. Goldman, L.A. Reduto, R.A. Langou, A. Gosttschalk and B.L. Zaret, 1979, *Am. J. Cardiol.*, 1159–1162.
89. Wallis, J.W., L. Wu-Connolly, A.P. Rocchine and J.E. Juni, 1986, *J. Nucl. Med.*, **27**, 1347–1352.
90. Boudraa, A., J.J. Mallet, J.E. Besson, S.E. Bouyoucef and J. Champier, 1993, *IEEE Trans. Med. Imaging*, **12**, 451–465.
91. Links, J.M., L.C. Becker, J.G. Shindledecker, P. Guzman, R.D. Burow, E.L. Nickoloff, P.O. Alderson and H.N. Wagner, 1982, *Circulation*, **65**, 82–91.
92. Massardo, T., R.A. Gal, R.P. Grenier, D.H. Schmidt and S.C. Port, 1990, *J. Nucl. Med.*, **31**, 450–456.
93. Gerbrands, J.J. and C. Hock, 1981, *Proc. 2nd. Int. Conf. Visual. Psychophys. Med. Imaging, Brussels, Belgium.* 155–159.
94. Goris, M.L., J.H. McKillop and P.A. Briandet, 1981, *Cardiovascular Int. Radiol.*, **4**, 117–123.
95. Duncan, J.S., 1987, *IEEE Trans. Med. Imaging*, **6**, 325–338.
96. Jouan, A., J. Verdenet, J.C. Cardot, M. Baud and J. Duvernoy, 1990, *IEEE Trans. Med. Imaging*, **9**, 5–10.
97. Boudraa, A., M. Arzi, J. Sau, J. Champier, S. Hadj-Moussa, J.E. Besson, D. Sapey-Marinier, R. Itti and J.J. Mallet, *IEEE Trans. Bimoed. Eng.* (In press).
98. Wagner, R.H., J.R. Halama, R.E. Henkin, G.L. Dillehay and P.A. Sobotka, 1989, *J. Nucl. Med.*, **30**, 1870–1874.
99. Underwood, S.R., S. Walton, P.J. Ell, P.H. Jarritt, R.W. Emanuel and R.M. Swanton, 1985, *Eur. J. Nucl. Med.*, **10**, 332–337.
100. Gill, J.B., R.H. Moore, N. Tamaki, D.D. Miller, M. Barlaikovach, T. Yasuda, C.A. Boucher and H.W. Strauss, 1986, *J. Nucl. Med.*, **27**, 1916–1920.
101. Callaham, R., J. Froelich, K. Mekusick, J. Leppo and H. Strauss, 1982, *J. Nucl. Med.*, **23**, 315–318.
102. Cerqueira, M.D., G.D. Harp and J.L. Ritchie, 1992, *J. Am. Coll. Cardiol.*, **20**, 934–941.
103. Faber, T.L., E.M. Stokely, G.H. Templeton, M.S. Akers, R.W. Parker and J.R. Corbett, 1989, *J. Nucl. Med.*, **30**, 638–649.
104. Faber, T.L., M.S. Akers, R.M. Peshock and J.R. Corbett, 1991, *J. Nucl. Med.*, **32**, 2311–2317.

105. Schelbert, H.R. and M. Schwaiger, 1986, In *Positron Emission Tomography and Autoradiography: Principles and Applications for the Brain and Heart* (E. Phelps, J.C. Mazziotta and H.R. Schelbet eds.) (Raven Press, New York), Chap. 12, pp. 581–661.
106. Higgins, C.B., W. Holt, P. Pflugfelder and U. Schtem, 1988, *Mag. Res. Med.*, **6**, 121–139.
107. Young, S.W., 1984, *Nuclear Magnetic Resonance Imaging: Basic Principles* (Raven Press, New York).
108. Chakeres, D.W. and P. Schmalbrock, 1992, *Fundamentals of Magnetic Resonance Imaging* (Williams and Wilkins, Baltimore).
109. Braunwald, E., 1992, *Heart Disease. A Textbook of Cardiovascular Medicine* (W.B. Saunders Company, Philadelphia), 4th ed., Chap. 11. pp. 312–341.
110. Acharya, R., R. Wasserman, J. Stevens and C. Hinojosa, 1995, *Comput. Med. Imag. Graph.*, **19**, 3–25.
111. Zerhouni, E.A., D.M. Parish, W.J. Rogers, A. Yang and E.P. Shapiro, 1988, *Radiology*, **169**, 59–63.
112. McVeigh, E.R. and E.A. Zerhouni, 1991, *Radiology*, **180**, 677–683.
113. Sechtem, U., P.W. Pflugfelder, R.D. White, R.G. Gould, W. Holt, M.J. Lipton and C.B. Higgins, 1987, *AJR*, **148**, 239–246.
114. Bezdek, J.C. and S.K. Pal, 1992, *Fuzzy Models For Pattern Recognition* (IEEE Press, New York).
115. Boudraa, A., J. Champier, Z. Hamici and J.J. Mallet, 1994, *Third Symposium on Medical Imaging Research, Paris, France*, 70.
116. Cohen, L.D., 1991, *CVGIP: Image Understanding*, **53**, 211–218.
117. Staib, L.H. and J.S. Duncan, 1992, *IEEE Trans. Pattern Anal. Machine Intell.*, **14**, 1061–1075.
118. Suhy, D.Y., R.L. Eisner, R.M. Mersereau and R.I. Pettigrew, 1993, *IEEE Trans. Med. Imaging*, **12**, 65–72.
119. Ranganath, S., 1995, *IEEE Trans. Med. Imaging*, **14**, 328–338.

3 TECHNIQUES IN IMAGE SEQUENCE FILTERING FOR CLINICAL ANGIOGRAPHY*

CHEUK L. CHAN,[1,†] A.K. KATSAGGELOS[2] and A.V. SAHAKIAN[2]

[1] *PAR Government Systems Corporation, 1010 Prospect Street, La Jolla, CA, 92037–4146, USA*
[2] *Department of Electrical Engineering and Computer Science, Northwestern University, Evanston, Illinois 60208-3118, USA*

3.1. INTRODUCTION

The assessment of coronary diseases through the evaluation of contrast imaging has been in existence for nearly a quarter century and has unquestionably aided physicians in their clinical exams. Of equal importance is a conscientious effort to reduce the risk factors of high X-ray exposure to both the patient and the medical staff. These two conflicting demands have often resulted in the degradation of image quality caused by the acquisition of radiographic images at low radiation levels. It is this noise that is treated here, since it has the greatest bearing on the tradeoff between radiation exposure and image quality. The aim of this chapter is to address this problem by first describing the process of radiation transport as a stochastic processs. Based on this description, a noise model is proposed from which a 3-D linear filter is derived to remove this noise. Its recursive counterpart is also presented here as a means of an efficient implementation. Finally, experimental results

---

*This research was supported in part by a grant from Siemens.

†C.L. Chan was with the Department of Electrical Engineering and Computer Science, Northwestern University, USA.

will be shown on clinical fluoroscopic images with both simulated and actual quantum mottle.

While both of these linear filters have given favorable results in terms of improving the image quality in mottled sequences, recent work in nonlinear filtering and simultaneous motion estimation and filtering may change the impetus of research in this area of clinical angiography. Some preliminary topics and results as they apply to this application will be pointed out in this chapter as well.

3.2. BACKGROUND

Historically, in digital subtraction angiography (DSA), vessels of interest were imaged by acquiring a series of X-ray images containing iodine contrast injected peripherally and subtracting them from a "mask" image of the same area obtained before opacification.[79] This noninvasive angiographic technique produces images suitable for diagnostic purposes if the structures of the mask image and contrast images are registered such as those found in renal or intracranial vasculatures. In addition, relatively low frame rate (1–2 frames/sec) image acquisitions (with a corresponding increase in exposure time) are possible for noncardiac applications if patient motion is limited. This increased radiation exposure (1 mR per frame) allows for improved contrast resolution and thus greater visibility of the area of interest.

More recently, particularly in cardiac applications, interest has focused on the use of selective intraarterial contrast administration (through the use of catheters) for the assessment of coronary disorders and visualization of higher order coronary branches. In these applications, the images are of sufficient high enough quality that image subtraction is not necessary. Correspondingly, frame rates are also higher for cardiac applications (30 frames/sec) since a longer pulse width such as that used in DSA would cause motion blurring of the vessels thus reducing the spatial resolution of the image.

Typically, for these cardiac applications, 100 to 200 frames are acquired at full radiographic levels for diagnosis (about 25 μR at the input of the image intensifier) integrating to a cumulative exposure of 3.8 mR to the image intensifier for 150 frames.[76] In addition, the guidance of the catheter to the coronary region requires occasional images to be acquired at fluoroscopic levels in those parts of the body where manipulation of the catheter is difficult. At these levels, quantum mottle is easily visible. Goldberg et al.,[35] have also considered the use of "boosted fluoroscopy" levels (i.e., tube current between fluoroscopic levels and full radiographic levels). These images may be sufficient for the location of stenotic regions as opposed to images acquired for quantitative coronary arteriography where full radiation levels are desirable. These different radiation levels have been developed for different tasks and the decision of which level to use has always been heavily weighed by the tradeoff of image quality versus patient safety. In addition, lower doses than these conventional levels may be desirable if post-processing of the images is possible.

Though the radiation can be lowered by acquiring frames at a lower rate (same pulse width and tube current as those in 30 frames/sec applications, but using a longer separation between pulses), objectionable flickering may result due to the jerkiness of the motion.[29] In addition, cardiologists often prefer a higher frame rate in order to have a sufficient number of points in the cardiac cycle, particularly near end diastole.[55]

A more preferable method of dosage reduction may be to vary the dosage from frame to frame. A group investigated this approach by varying the intensity between two extreme levels (0.5 and 10 mAs), allowing high X-ray intensities for periods of maximum and minimum opacification of the vessel and low X-ray intensities in between.[67]

Enzmann et al.[23] proposed low-dose, high-frame-rate versus regular dose, low-frame-rate subtraction angiography at the same X-ray tube voltage. However, their work was with dosages in the vicinity of 200 μR (i.e., generator parameters of 75–90 kV and 300 mA at 4–7 frames per second), which is considerably higher than the range of exposures considered in this chapter. Despite this difference, they found that low-dose techniques can be successful in cases where patient motion is limited during the data acquisition process. When this case is true, low-dose fluoroscopy can generate very accurate information regarding the iodination of the arteries of interest.

The goal in low-dose fluoroscopy and low-dose angiography is to pursue this idea of continuous variability of X-ray dosage levels from frame to frame. By increasing the exposure during relevant frames and similarly by decreasing it during less relevant frames, it is possible to effectively administer X-ray dosage levels satisfactory to both the patient's risk and image quality. Relevant frames refers to those frames where there is considerable motion, nonlinear motion, or occlusions that a post processing algorithm such as image sequence filtering which filters multiple images by using motion estimation techniques cannot handle, or considerable noise which is not created as a direct result of the exposure level (e.g., camera noise which may arise from a sudden saturation). During the less relevant frames, filtering techniques may be employed to enhance mottle-corrupted images that would naturally arise with a dosage reduction. Before these methods can be discussed, it is necessary to mathematically characterize the phenomenon of a reduced radiation exposure and to describe its effects on image quality.

3.3. NOISE MODELING

It is well known that the emission of photons from an X-ray source can be described by a Poisson process.[57] When the number of photons available for imaging is limited, such as in the case of low-dose fluoroscopy, quantum noise caused by the discretization of energy into photons becomes more evident. This noise manifests itself as a granularity in the image due to statistical fluctuations in the arrival of X-ray photons at the image intensifier.[9] In general, this statistical fluctuation varies in both space and time and constitutes a doubly stochastic Poisson point process[10,26,75] with a spatially and temporally varying intensity function. Therefore, the noise statistics may change both spatially, from pixel to pixel, and temporally, from frame to frame depending on the intensity at that particular location. This is consistent with the notion of quantum and/or signal-dependent noise.

In this chapter, the discussion will be limited to minimum mean square error (MMSE) filtering techniques. For these techniques, it is useful to describe an additive noise model

$$\mathbf{g}_i(\mathbf{r}) = \mathbf{f}_i(\mathbf{r}) + \mathbf{n}_i(\mathbf{r}) \tag{1}$$

where $\mathbf{f}$ is the true, unknown signal, $\mathbf{g}$ is the observed, degraded signal and $\mathbf{n}$ is the signal-dependent noise term. The spatial index, $\mathbf{r}$, and the temporal index, i, indicate the spatial and temporal dependency of each term.

Without loss of generality, the observed degraded images are related to the observed counting processes, $\mathbf{N}$, at the image intensifier through a scale factor, λ,

$$\mathbf{g}_i(\mathbf{r}) = \frac{1}{\lambda}\mathbf{N}_i(\mathbf{r}), \tag{2}$$

where $\mathbf{N}_i$ has a Poisson probability density function (pdf) when conditioned on the intensity $\mathbf{f}$,

$$p(\mathbf{N}_i|\mathbf{f}) = \prod_{\mathbf{r}\in A} p(\mathbf{N}_i(\mathbf{r}) = m_r|\mathbf{f}(\mathbf{r}))$$

$$= \prod_{\mathbf{r}\in A} [\lambda\mathbf{f}(\mathbf{r})]^{m_r} \exp\{-\lambda\mathbf{f}(\mathbf{r})\}/m_r!,$$

for the image plane A, as shown in Figure 1. The term, m_r, represents the observed counts at pixel location $\mathbf{r}$ in frame i. Therefore, the displayed image

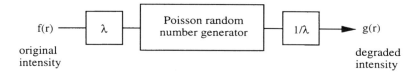

Figure 1. Poisson noise simulator, after [60].

intensity, $g(\mathbf{r})$, has the conditional pdf

$$p_{\mathbf{g}}(\mathbf{g}_i(\mathbf{r})|\mathbf{f}_i(\mathbf{r})) = \lambda p(\lambda \mathbf{g}_i(\mathbf{r})|\mathbf{f}_i(\mathbf{r}))$$

$$= \lambda \frac{(\lambda \mathbf{f}_i(\mathbf{r}))^{\lambda \mathbf{g}_i(\mathbf{r})} e^{-\lambda \mathbf{f}_i(\mathbf{r})}}{\left[\lambda \mathbf{g}_i(\mathbf{r})\right]!}. \tag{3}$$

The mean and variance of the quantum noise, $\mathbf{n}(\mathbf{r})$, in Equation (1) can thus be shown to be [11,54]

$$E\{\mathbf{n}(\mathbf{r})\} = 0$$

$$\sigma_{\mathbf{n}}^2(\mathbf{r}) = \frac{1}{\lambda} E\{\mathbf{f}(\mathbf{r})\}. \tag{4}$$

In addition, the 3rd and 4th order moments of this noise is given by (see Appendix)

$$E\{\mathbf{n}^3(\mathbf{r})\} = \frac{1}{\lambda^2} E\{\mathbf{f}(\mathbf{r})\}$$

$$E\{\mathbf{n}^4(\mathbf{r})\} = \frac{1}{\lambda^3} E\{\mathbf{f}(\mathbf{r})\} + \frac{3}{\lambda^2} E\{\mathbf{f}^2(r)\}.$$

These higher order moments are useful for nonlinear MMSE filtering of images containing quantum noise,[17] as this quantum noise cannot be uniquely characterized by the 1st and 2nd order moments alone as in Gaussian noise. These moments will be useful for the discussion of the nonlinear filter in Section 3.7. It can be shown,[75] that the additive noise model in Equation (1) leads to an equivalent integral equation for the solution of the optimum linear estimate as that obtained if the conditional pdf in Equation (3) is used, thus justifying the formulation of such a model. Now that a model for the quantum mottle has been presented, several methods of filtering image sequences based on this model can and will be formulated in Section 3.5. First, however, a review of image sequence filtering and motion estimation is warranted.

3.4. IMAGE SEQUENCE FILTERING

3.4.1. Filtering

Various filtering methods have been proposed in the past to remove noise in X-ray images. Traditionally, these methods did not assume a model for the noise and thus could not be assessed in terms of any optimality criteria other than a visual comparison.[25,37] Furthermore, these methods neglect to treat the specific problem of noise arising from a reduction of radiation level (e.g., quantum mottle).

Though not specifically applied to the clinical arena, several methods for filtering single frame photon-limited scenes have been proposed in the past. Kuan et al.,[54] derived a linear nonstationary minimum mean square error (MMSE) method for filtering signal-dependent noise. Poisson distributed quantum-limited noise can be seen to belong in this more general class of noise since the fluctuation of photons is directly proportional to the number of photons available in the signal (see Equation (4)). Kasturi et al.,[48] through independent work, also arrived at a Bayesian estimator for treating signal-dependent noise, but taking into account the presence of additive white Gaussian noise as well in their observation equation. Jiang and Sawchuk[45] expanded on Kuan's filter by proposing to iteratively smooth a degraded image containing signal-dependent noise. Their technique also involves repeatedly updating the covariance matrix to reflect the reduction in noise levels in the image after each filtering stage. In these Bayesian techniques, different methods were used to obtain the *a priori* probabilities needed in the formulation of the estimators. For example, Kuan et al.,[54] and Jiang and Sawchuk[45] used local statistics to estimate the *a priori* densities of the image. This led to the nonstationary filters that they derived. Kasturi et al.,[48] used a Gaussian and Laplacian model for their work. Hull et al.,[42] also proposed a Bayesian approach for nuclear medicine image data, but obtained the necessary *a priori* probabilities from a clinical ensemble of past patient studies. Finally, Frieden[27] derived a Maximum *a posteriori* (MAP) method for severely quantum limited images (e.g., astronomical images) wherein the noise statistics are governed by a negative binomial distribution rather than a Poisson distribution because the quantum degeneracy factor is not negligible for these types of images.

Nevertheless, given a sequence of photon-limited images, these methods would individually filter each frame independently of all other frames in the sequence without taking advantage of any temporal correlations between frames — a factor that can significantly enhance filter performance. It has been shown that simple averaging along the time axis is not an effective form of temporal processing in dynamic sequences as it tends to blur moving objects[20,47] Even if these images are first registered and then averaged, the development of a model for the noise, based on physical principles, leads to a better filter, in terms of performance. Instead, the filtering of image sequences can be placed into a different class of problems.

Specifically, image sequence filtering may be classified into two categories: motion compensated and non-motion compensated. Non-motion compensated temporal filters address only the problem of estimating the intensity field by assuming that little or no motion has occurred between frames. There are two general forms of non-motion compensated temporal filters, depending on the number of filtered estimates desired. A single filtered estimate recovered from a set of observations could be obtained from a *multiple-input filter*, whereas simultaneous restoration of all the frames in a set of observations leading to multiple filtered estimates can be obtained through a *multi-channel filter*.

Ghiglia[34] first addressed the problem of multiple input image restoration by considering N independently blurred images of a common object. He implemented a constrained least-squares filter in the frequency domain similar in form to the Wiener filter. Katsaggelos[49] also treated this problem by using a set-theoretic approach to arrive at a least-squares solution. Hunt and Kubler[43] treat the restoration of color images as a multi-channel image restoration problem. Using the MMSE criterion, they derived a multi-channel filter based on the assumption that the multispectral components can be separated through a Karhunen-Loeve transform. After this decorrelation, the images are filtered individually with a single frame Wiener filter. Galatsanos *et al.*,[30,31] tackle the multichannel image restoration problem directly by taking into consideration cross-channel correlations without using the separability assumption and develop a multiframe Wiener restoration algorithm.

Motion compensated temporal filters, on the other hand, utilize cross-correlations along the direction of motion. However this requires the estimation of the displacement vector field (DVF) from the noisy frames. Nevertheless, when it is available, or it can be estimated, a motion compensated temporal filter can be seen to belong in the class of multiple input filters. Huang and Tsai[41] proposed one of the first techniques by doing simple averaging of the frames. For the reasons mentioned earlier, however, averaging of the frames is not an effective form of temporal processing. Dubois and Sabri[20] first looked at image sequence filtering for a videoconferencing application by proposing a nonlinear recursive filter to operate on motion compensated frames. Because the motion estimator they used did not take into account the presence of noise, the results were not as good for the very noisy environments as for low noise environments. To combat this problem, Katsaggelos *et al.*,[50] proposed a 3-D separable recursive motion-compensated spatio-temporal filter to utilize correlations not just in the temporal domain but also correlations in the spatial domain as well. The correlation coefficients were calculated for the steady state case, thus assuming that the image intensity field is stationary. To avoid this problem, an edge adaptive motion compensated spatio-temporal filter was proposed in [51], where the response of the filter is tuned to spatial edge information and motion compensation prediction error. Now, however, the performance of their estimator, is also tied to the performance of the edge detector in noisy environments. Brailean and Katsaggelos[5,6] have proposed a novel method for filtering image sequences in additive white Gaussian noise (AWGN) by proposing a robust motion estimator that performs well in noisy environments. In addition, an extended Kalman filter is used to filter the motion compensated image sequence. Both estimators are based on the use of doubly stochastic Markov models driven by a Gibbs distribution[33] for the expression of the motion and intensity field.[7]

All of these image sequence filtering techniques described thus far have been formulated for sequences degraded by AWGN. Although these methods may arguably be applied to the problem at hand, they cannot correctly model the underlying quantum–limited imaging processes. For example, Singh[72] used a recursive technique to perform motion-compensated enhancement of cardiac fluoroscopy image sequences. His technique follows from an incremental Kalman filtering-based method for estimating the motion field and the intensity field separately. Though he obtained good results on clinical sequences simulated with white Gaussian noise, Singh discussed the fact that X-ray images are known to have signal-dependent Poisson noise and that there is a need for temporal versions of filters for these types of noise.

3.4.2. Motion Estimation

While there have been numerous algorithms for registering angiographic images (see, for example, [78,79]), these methods assume that there is no noise in the images. The estimation of the DVF by specifically taking into consideration the presence of noise have only recently been considered, with the majority of the work confined to the additive white Gaussian noise (AWGN) environment. The beginnings of these works resulted primarily in maximum likelihood approaches to estimate the motion field whereby Gaussian assumptions are made to make the problem more tractable.[58,61,64] Anderson and Giannakis[2] considered the use of higher order cumulants for estimating the DVF in correlated Gaussian noise. Abdelqader and Rajala[1] took into consideration *a priori* knowledge of the motion field by using Gibbs distribution and applying a mean field annealing technique to noisy sequences in order to obtain the result. Konrad and Dubois[53] also used a Gibbs distribution in their characterization of the DVF, but solved for the solution using MAP and minimum expected cost methods. Brailean and Katsaggelos[7] treated the problem recursively and obtained MAP estimates of the motion field from noisy sequences using an extended Kalman filter.

These approaches preclude those techniques which treat the motion field as an observed noisy signal requiring post-processing. In the application to quantum-limited scenes, Pohlig[70] investigated the detection of moving optical targets from a CCD sensor in Poisson noise, but does not consider the estimation problem. Though Chen[18] extends this detection problem further to account for three-dimensional moving targets, the *estimation* of the DVF by specifically taking into consideration the presence of noise have only recently been considered, with the majority of the work confined to the additive white Gaussian noise environment. Morris[62] describes a method for scene matching using photon-limited images, but assumes the availability of an original reference scene for cross-correlation against the degraded frame. In general, the two frames of a dynamic sequence, such as those considered here, are both degraded and the original reference frame is not available. Chan and Katsaggelos[16] have proposed an iterative method for estimating DVF's from quantum-limited scenes. This approach will be described in Section 3.8. In addition, Chan *et al.*,[8,15] extend this method further by considering the use of a Gibbs distribution to describe the motion field to improve upon the estimates.

In general, the registration of images in noise through motion compensation is a difficult problem. Consequently, in order for image sequence filtering to be optimal, the two tasks of displacement field estimation and image enhancement should be treated simultaneously as was done in [15,16]. In the first part of this chapter, image sequence filtering in quantum-limited noise is treated as a two-stage problem instead; that is, the estimation of the displacement field is treated separately from the estimation of the image intensity field. Although this may not provide the best possible results, separability enables a simpler, yet more insightful, formulation of the problem, while still yielding improved estimates over spatial filtering alone. Later, in Section 3.8, some preliminary work on the simultaneous motion estimation and filtering approach will be presented for the quantum-limited case.

Perfect registration of two frames, $\mathbf{f_1}$ and $\mathbf{f_2}$, undergoing purely translational motion implies that $\mathbf{f} \stackrel{\text{def}}{=} \mathbf{f_2}(\mathbf{r}) = \mathbf{f_1}(\mathbf{r} - \mathbf{d}(\mathbf{r}))$, where $\mathbf{d}$ is the spatially and temporally varying DVF. The commonly made assumptions of constant brightness and no occlusions of moving objects are made here. In practice, $\mathbf{f_1}$ and $\mathbf{f_2}$ are not available for motion compensation. Therefore, the degraded observations, $\mathbf{g_1}$ and $\mathbf{g_2}$, must be used to obtain the motion vector estimates.

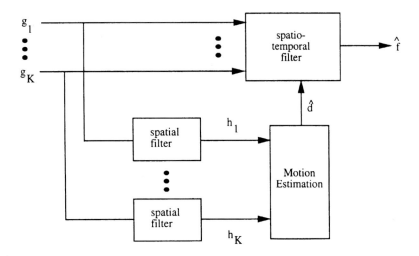

Figure 2. Block diagram of motion-compensated temporal filter.

Such an implementation is shown in Figure 2. Katsaggelos *et al.*[50] have shown that with noise above a certain level, registration errors become so large that it is necessary to spatially filter each frame separately before motion estimation can be performed. This is also true for the clinical fluoroscopic image sequences shown in this chapter. This optional step is also shown in Figure 2.

It is important to note that displacement estimates obtained with this spatial filtering preprocessing stage are used for the temporal filtering of the *degraded* frames, and *not* the spatially filtered frames. The latter procedure of applying the temporal filter to the spatially filtered frames may result in the oversmoothing of the image causing edges to become blurred. This "iterative" filtering (so named because of applying filtering to the degraded images and then to the newly filtered image again) was implemented with Kuan's spatial filter, as mentioned earlier, in [45]. It entails updating the noise covariance matrix in the original formulation to reflect the presence of new noise levels after spatial filtering once. While this approach is not addressed here, an application of a temporal version of this "iterative" filter to angiographic image sequences can be found in [14].

Next, a method is described for obtaining an estimate of the vector field, **d**, between $\mathbf{g_1}$ and $\mathbf{g_2}$, or their spatially filtered counterparts, $\mathbf{h_1}$ and $\mathbf{h_2}$. Two different approaches have been implemented in this study

— namely, a block matching algorithm using an exhaustive mean square matching criterion[65] and a Wiener-based pel-recursive algorithm[4,21,22] with similar filtering results. Block matching algorithms constitute shifting image subblocks between two frames to find the direction of maximum correlation. Pel (or pixel) recursive algorithms recursively compute a displacement vector for each pixel using gradient-based minimization.[65] Generally, block matching algorithms are more robust to large displacements in the sequence, although the DVF produces noticeably more blocking artifacts, when used for compensation of the motion. However, this problem can be compensated for by choosing overlapping blocks and interpolating the vectors away from the center of the block. Because the fluoroscopic sequence used in the simulations may contain displacements of as much as 10 pixels between two consecutive frames, the block matching algorithm described above was used to obtain the DVF. For even larger displacements, a bigger search space may be used in the block matching algorithm. Alternatively, the radiation dosage may be raised at this point in anticipation of the jump in motion, in essence, turning off the temporal filter. Some *a priori* information must be utilized regarding the structure being imaged to determine whether the displacement is beyond the specifications of the motion estimation algorithm.

In the next section, a 3-D locally linear minimum mean square error (LLMMSE) filter is derived based on the noise model discussed in Section 3.3. This filter will operate on a set of registered images obtained through the motion estimation algorithm just discussed.

3.5. 3-D LLMMSE FILTER

The proposed 3-D linear minimum mean square error (LMMSE) filter is derived in this section for the multiple-input case, which assumes the availability of a set of motion compensated frames degraded by quantum-limited noise. As discussed in the previous section, this set of registered frames is obtained separately by using a DVF which was obtained independently.

3.5.1. Filter Formulation

Consider the lexicographically ordered representation of the set of observation equations given by

$$\mathbf{g}_i = \mathbf{f}_i + \mathbf{n}_i, \qquad i = 1, \ldots, K, \qquad (6)$$

where $\mathbf{g}_i$ is the i-th observation vector, representing the lexicographically ordered i-th degraded frame, $\mathbf{f}_i$ is the i-th original image, and $\mathbf{n}_i$ is the i-th zero-mean signal-dependent noise vector, uncorrelated with $\mathbf{n}_j$ for $i \neq j$. Furthermore, each original frame is compensated to the K-th original frame through a set of displacement vectors such that

$$f_i(\mathbf{r} - \mathbf{d}_{i,K}(\mathbf{r})) = f_K(\mathbf{r}),$$

$\forall \mathbf{r} = 1, \ldots, M^2$ and $\forall i = 1, \ldots, K - 1$, where $\mathbf{d}_{i,K}(\mathbf{r})$ is the spatially varying displacement vector relating the intensity in frame i to frame K at spatial location $\mathbf{r}$. Furthermore, let the motion compensated frames representing the observation and noise images be denoted by

$$\mathbf{g}_i^{MC} \overset{\text{def}}{=} \mathbf{g}_i(\underline{\mathbf{r}} - \underline{\mathbf{d}}_{i,K})$$

$$\mathbf{n}_i^{MC} \overset{\text{def}}{=} \mathbf{n}_i(\underline{\mathbf{r}} - \underline{\mathbf{d}}_{i,K})$$

and the motion compensated original image by

$$\mathbf{f} \overset{\text{def}}{=} \mathbf{f}_K.$$

Consequently, Equation (6) may be rewritten as

$$\mathbf{g}_i^{MC} = \mathbf{f} + \mathbf{n}_i^{MC}, \qquad i = 1, \ldots, K - 1,$$

and

$$\mathbf{g}_K = \mathbf{f} + \mathbf{n}_K.$$

For ease of notation, these vectors are further stacked into a single observation equation resulting in

$$\underline{\mathbf{g}} = \underline{\mathbf{f}} + \underline{\mathbf{n}}, \tag{7}$$

where

$$\underline{\mathbf{g}} = \begin{bmatrix} \mathbf{g}_1^{MC} \\ \mathbf{g}_2^{MC} \\ \vdots \\ \mathbf{g}_K \end{bmatrix}$$

and similarly for $\underline{\mathbf{f}}$ and $\underline{\mathbf{n}}$. All the vectors, $\underline{\mathbf{g}}$, $\underline{\mathbf{f}}$, and $\underline{\mathbf{n}}$, are of dimensions $KM^2 \times 1$.

Using the additive signal-dependent noise model derived in Section 3.3, a minimum mean square error estimate is sought which minimizes the mean square prediction error,

$$E\{(\underline{\mathbf{f}} - \hat{\underline{\mathbf{f}}})^2\}.$$

The optimal estimate, $\hat{\underline{\mathbf{f}}}$, is given by the conditional mean [66]

$$\hat{\underline{\mathbf{f}}} = E\{\underline{\mathbf{f}}|\mathbf{g}_1^{MC}, \mathbf{g}_2^{MC}, \ldots, \mathbf{g}_K\}.$$

In general, this conditional mean is nonlinear. However, it was pointed out in Section 3.3 and shown in [75] that the use of an additive noise model leads to an equivalent integral equation for the solution of the optimum linear estimate as that obtained if the conditional mean was constrained to be linear. In other words, the formulation of an additive noise model from the Poisson data allows one to approximate the conditional mean with a linear estimator of the form

$$\hat{\underline{\mathbf{f}}} = \Gamma_0 \mathbf{1} + \Gamma_1 \mathbf{g}_1^{MC} + \cdots + \Gamma_K \mathbf{g}_K, \qquad (8)$$

where $\mathbf{1}$ is a vector of KM^2 1's, and the Γ_i's are matrices of dimensions KM^2 by M^2 containing the unknown coefficients to be determined. The optimal linear estimate is given by the multichannel LMMSE filter

$$\hat{\underline{\mathbf{f}}} = E\{\underline{\mathbf{f}}\} + \mathbf{C}_{\underline{\mathbf{f}}\,\underline{\mathbf{g}}} \mathbf{C}_{\underline{\mathbf{g}}\,\underline{\mathbf{g}}}^{-1} \left[\underline{\mathbf{g}} - E\{\underline{\mathbf{g}}\}\right], \qquad (9)$$

which is similar to the single-channel LMMSE estimator[54,66], where $\mathbf{C}_{\underline{\mathbf{f}}\,\underline{\mathbf{g}}}$ is the cross-covariance matrix and $\mathbf{C}_{\underline{\mathbf{g}}\,\underline{\mathbf{g}}}$ is the covariance matrix. It should be noted that this filter is different from the multichannel Wiener filter in [43,30], because of the nonstationarity involved. For example, the matrix $\mathbf{C}_{\underline{\mathbf{g}}\,\underline{\mathbf{g}}}$ is not block circulant and therefore fast Fourier transform (FFT) techniques cannot be used to obtain its inverse, and all operations are performed in the spatial domain.

Because the $\underline{\mathbf{f}}$ vector consists of K identically stacked versions of $\mathbf{f}$, Equation (9) is simplified to a multiple-input LMMSE filter

$$\hat{\mathbf{f}} = E\{\mathbf{f}\} + \mathbf{C}_{\mathbf{f}\,\underline{\mathbf{g}}} \mathbf{C}_{\underline{\mathbf{g}}\,\underline{\mathbf{g}}}^{-1} \left[\underline{\mathbf{g}} - E\{\underline{\mathbf{g}}\}\right], \qquad (10)$$

where $\mathbf{C_{f\underline{g}}} = \left[\mathbf{C}_{\mathbf{f}g_1^{MC}} \vdots \mathbf{C}_{\mathbf{f}g_2^{MC}} \vdots \cdots \vdots \mathbf{C}_{\mathbf{f}g_K} \right]$. Expanding the terms, Equation (10) becomes

$$\hat{\mathbf{f}} = E\{\mathbf{f}\}+ \tag{11}$$

$$\begin{bmatrix} \mathbf{C}_{\mathbf{f}g_1^{MC}} \\ \mathbf{C}_{\mathbf{f}g_2^{MC}} \\ \vdots \\ \mathbf{C}_{\mathbf{f}g_K} \end{bmatrix}^T \begin{bmatrix} \mathbf{C}_{g_1^{MC}g_1^{MC}} & \mathbf{C}_{g_1^{MC}g_2^{MC}} & \cdots & \mathbf{C}_{g_1^{MC}g_K} \\ \mathbf{C}_{g_2^{MC}g_1^{MC}} & \mathbf{C}_{g_2^{MC}g_2^{MC}} & \cdots & \mathbf{C}_{g_2^{MC}g_K} \\ \vdots & & & \\ \mathbf{C}_{g_Kg_1^{MC}} & \mathbf{C}_{g_Kg_2^{MC}} & \cdots & \mathbf{C}_{g_Kg_K} \end{bmatrix}^{-1} \begin{bmatrix} g_1^{MC} - E\{g_1^{MC}\} \\ g_2^{MC} - E\{g_2^{MC}\} \\ \vdots \\ g_K - E\{g_K\} \end{bmatrix},$$

where all the submatrices are diagonal, thus making $\mathbf{C_{\underline{g}\ \underline{g}}}$ a sub-block diagonal matrix. The similarity between this multiple-input filter and the multichannel filter in Equation (9) is evident because $\mathbf{f}_1, \mathbf{f}_2, \ldots, \mathbf{f}_{K-1}$ are all related to $\mathbf{f}_K$ through the respective DVF's. In this instance, the solution for all the motion-compensated channels of the multichannel filter is identical to the solution for a single channel, as given by the multiple-input filter.

In Equation (11), the inversion of $\mathbf{C_{\underline{g}\ \underline{g}}}$, of dimensions $KM^2 \times KM^2$, is required. Even for moderate size images, ($M = 256$), this inversion is unmanageable. However, the matrix is sub-block diagonal due to the nonstationary mean nonstationary variance (NMNV) assumption of no correlation between pixels, and therefore, it is a straightforward task to perform the inversion. It can be shown that the inverse has the same sub-block diagonal form and that the inversion of this KM^2 by KM^2 sub-block diagonal matrix can be decomposed into M^2 inversions of K by K matrices.[31] In other words, there exist M^2 locally linear MMSE (LLMMSE) separate filters, one for each pixel. This seems reasonable, since the intensity of $\mathbf{f}$ is actually a mixture of Gaussians, with nonstationary means and nonstationary variances.

The term *local* refers to the neighborhood around the working pixel in which the spatially varying means and variances of the NMNV model are estimated. Specifically, since the means and variances vary from pixel to pixel and the pixels are jointly independent, each filter at a spatial location $\mathbf{r}$ operates independently of the filters at other spatial locations. Furthermore, the estimation of these nonstationary first and second order moments is also done locally — within a local spatial analysis window. A larger window can give a more accurate estimate of these statistics provided that there are no edges in the window. The presence of discontinuities can cause undesirable biases in these estimates. With motion-compensated image sequences, however, there exists K realizations of the random field. Therefore, the spatial dimensions of these local windows can be made smaller than their counterparts in the still frame case, while still providing good estimates since multiple frames are used, and the temporal dimension of these windows is greater than one.

With the above assumptions, the LLMMSE filter takes the following form at each pixel[11]:

$$\hat{f}(\mathbf{r}) = \bar{f}(\mathbf{r}) + \begin{bmatrix} v_{fg_1^{MC}}(\mathbf{r}) \\ v_{fg_2^{MC}}(\mathbf{r}) \\ \vdots \\ v_{fg_K}(\mathbf{r}) \end{bmatrix}^T \tag{12}$$

$$\cdot \begin{bmatrix} v_{g_1^{MC}g_1^{MC}}(\mathbf{r}) & v_{g_1^{MC}g_2^{MC}}(\mathbf{r}) & \cdots & v_{g_1^{MC}g_K}(\mathbf{r}) \\ v_{g_2^{MC}g_1^{MC}}(\mathbf{r}) & v_{g_2^{MC}g_2^{MC}}(\mathbf{r}) & \cdots & v_{g_2^{MC}g_K}(\mathbf{r}) \\ & \vdots & & \\ v_{g_Kg_1^{MC}}(\mathbf{r}) & v_{g_Kg_2^{MC}}(\mathbf{r}) & \cdots & v_{g_Kg_K}(\mathbf{r}) \end{bmatrix}^{-1} \begin{bmatrix} g_1^{MC}(\mathbf{r}) - \bar{g}_1^{MC}(\mathbf{r}) \\ g_2^{MC}(\mathbf{r}) - \bar{g}_2^{MC}(\mathbf{r}) \\ \vdots \\ g_K(\mathbf{r}) - \bar{g}_K(\mathbf{r})\} \end{bmatrix},$$

where $v_{fg_i}(\mathbf{r}) = \sigma^2_{fg_i}(\mathbf{r})$, $v_{g_ig_j}(\mathbf{r}) = \sigma^2_{g_ig_j}(\mathbf{r})$ are the local variances, and $\bar{f}(\mathbf{r})$, and $\bar{g}(\mathbf{r})$ represent the corresponding local means of $f(\mathbf{r})$ and $g(\mathbf{r})$. It is interesting to note that when $K = 1$, the filter in Equation (12) is similar to the spatial filter for single images developed by Kuan et al. in [54]. For the single-frame case, the local cross-covariance, $\sigma^2_{fg}(\mathbf{r})$, can be shown to be equal to the local variance of $f(\mathbf{r})$, or $\sigma^2_f(\mathbf{r})$. Then, the inversion of each K by K matrix is replaced by a scalar in the denominator leading to M^2 expressions, one for each pixel, for the estimate of the original image

$$\hat{f}(\mathbf{r}) = \bar{f}(\mathbf{r}) + \frac{\sigma^2_f(\mathbf{r})}{\sigma^2_g(\mathbf{r})} [g(\mathbf{r}) - \bar{g}(\mathbf{r})], \qquad \mathbf{r} = 1 \ldots M^2,$$

which is identical to Equation (17) in Kuan's paper.[54]

To see the properties of the temporal filter, it is useful to consider the case of 2 frames. That is, when $K = 2$, the filter in Equation (12) simplifies to:

$$\hat{f}(\mathbf{r}) = E\{f(\mathbf{r})\} + \beta_1(\mathbf{r}) \left[g_1^{MC}(\mathbf{r}) - E\{g_1^{MC}(\mathbf{r})\}\right]$$
$$+ \beta_2(\mathbf{r}) [g_2(\mathbf{r}) - E\{g_2(\mathbf{r})\}] \mathbf{r} = 1 \ldots M^2, \tag{13}$$

where the optimal coefficients $\beta_1(\mathbf{r})$ and $\beta_2(\mathbf{r})$ are determined by performing M^2 inversions of size 2 by 2 matrices, thus leading to

$$\beta_1(\mathbf{r}) = \frac{\sigma_{n_2}^2(\mathbf{r})\sigma_f^2(\mathbf{r})}{\sigma_f^2(\mathbf{r})\left[\sigma_{n_1}^2(\mathbf{r}) + \sigma_{n_2}^2(\mathbf{r})\right] + \sigma_{n_1}^2(\mathbf{r})\sigma_{n_2}^2(\mathbf{r})},$$

$$\beta_2(\mathbf{r}) = \frac{\sigma_{n_1}^2(\mathbf{r})\sigma_f^2(\mathbf{r})}{\sigma_f^2(\mathbf{r})\left[\sigma_{n_1}^2(\mathbf{r}) + \sigma_{n_2}^2(\mathbf{r})\right] + \sigma_{n_1}^2(\mathbf{r})\sigma_{n_2}^2(\mathbf{r})}.$$

(14)

In accordance with the discussion in Section 3.2, this filter is more versatile to the low-dose fluoroscopy situation where the noise may change levels from frame to frame than a technique which reduces dosage through frame-interpolation algorithms. Some insight into the filter's performance may be gained upon closer examination of Equation (13). For example, if frame 1 is much noisier than frame 2 (i.e., $\beta_2 >> \beta_1$), then the second observation is weighted more in the filter. Likewise, if frame 2 is noisier than frame 1 (i.e., $\beta_1 >> \beta_2$), then frame 1 is weighted more than frame 2. Finally, if both frames 1 and 2 are very noisy (i.e., $\beta_1 + \beta_2 << 1$), then the mean of $f(\mathbf{r})$ becomes a better estimate.

In the development of the temporal filter, it is noted that although an arbitrary number of frames may be used as input, rarely will more than 3 frames ever be used. This is limited primarily by the accuracy of the motion estimation stage since scene changes and/or occlusions will inevitably be encountered after a significant number of frames in any sequence. Here, an interleaved approach is used to recover each frame whereby the filter operates on no more than 3 frames at a time and moves on to the next temporal location upon completion. A more efficient approach may be to recursively estimate subsequent frames utilizing new information in an intuitive manner as shown in Section 3.6. In the next section, the performance of the 3-D LLMMSE filter on clinical image sequences corrupted with simulated quantum mottle is shown.

3.5.2. Experimental Results

In this section, the multiple-input filter, as given by Equation (12), is experimentally compared on a segment of a clinical image sequence simulated with various levels of Poisson-distributed noise, typical of quantum-limited images when the dosage is significantly reduced. Some indication of the amount of motion present in the sequence is shown in Figure 3. Here, the mean square frame difference (MSFD) of the original intensities between frames k and $k-1$ of dimensions M^2 is given by

$$\text{MSFD}(k) = \frac{1}{M^2}\sum_{\mathbf{r}}\left[f_k(\mathbf{r}) - f_{k-1}(\mathbf{r})\right]^2.$$

(15)

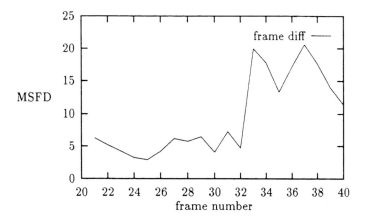

Figure 3. Mean square frame difference of image sequence.

In this sequence, periods of both low and heavy motion, as reflected by the MSFD figure, are shown in Figure 3.

The performance of the filter is evaluated over the entire sequence with the same simulated dosage and is measured by the improvement in the signal-to-noise ratio in dB per frame:

$$I_{SNR}(k) = 10 \log_{10} \frac{\sum_{\mathbf{r}} [g_k(\mathbf{r}) - f_k(\mathbf{r})]^2}{\sum_{\mathbf{r}} \left[\hat{f}_k(\mathbf{r}) - f_k(\mathbf{r}) \right]^2}. \tag{16}$$

The average improvement in signal to noise ratio, $\bar{I}_{SNR}$, over N frames of the sequence is given by

$$\bar{I}_{SNR} = \frac{1}{N} \sum_{k=1}^{N} I_{SNR}(k).$$

Motion blocks of size 16×16 and a maximum search space of 10 pixels in either direction were used. In addition, overlapping blocks were used to provide a denser displacement vector field.

Table 1 compares the average improvement in SNR, $\bar{I}_{SNR}$, for the temporal filters versus Kuan's spatial filter averaged over 20 different frames of the same fluoroscopic sequence at the same dosage. The window size reflects the dimensions of the spatial window used to obtain the local statistics around the working pixel. Note that, in general, the multiple-input filters increase in

Table 1. $\bar{I}_{SNR}$ (in dB) for a 20-frame segment of fluoro sequence.

λ	window size	spatial filtering 2-D Kuan	temporal filtering 3-D MC LLMMSE 2-frames	3-frames
.25	5×5	11.68	14.39	15.46
.50	5×5	11.42	13.84	14.48
.75	5×5	11.21	13.43	13.74
.25	7×7	13.94	16.27	16.90
.50	7×7	13.32	15.28	15.46
.75	7×7	12.83	14.54	14.45

performance with increasing noise (i.e., decreasing values of λ), since there is room for greater improvement in the noisier images.

Figure 4 shows the performance of each filter on a per-frame basis at λ = 0.5 for the window size of 7 × 7 pixels used to compute the local statistics. Note that the three-frame temporal filter performs better than the two-frame temporal filter and the spatial filter in areas of the sequence with low to moderate motion, but suffers somewhat when reconstructing those frames with considerable motion as in frames 32–40 in Figure 3. This may be attributed to the fact that the motion is not necessarily linear across three frames in addition to the inability of the motion estimator to track the vessel across more than two frames. During the latter frames of the sequence, the performance of the motion-compensated filters become particularly sensitive to the fluctuations from frame to frame.

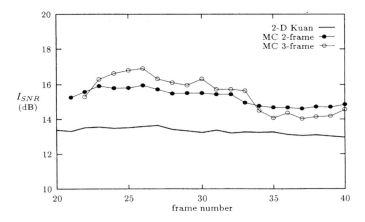

Figure 4. $I_{SNR}(k)$ for fluoro sequence, 7 × 7 window, λ = 0.50.

Table 1 demonstrates precisely the tradeoff of increasing the temporal support at the expense of decreasing the size of the analysis window. For example, a 2-frame temporal filter gives a 14.39 dB SNR improvement for a 5 × 5 window versus a single frame filter which gives about the same (13.94 dB) improvement for a bigger window size of 7 × 7 pixels. The advantages of decreasing the size of the spatial analysis window includes a reduction in the computational load as well as in the chances of smoothing out object boundaries. Therefore, a similar increase in the temporal support from one frame to two frames (or from two frames to three frames) does not significantly increase the computational burden since the size of the matrices to be inverted only increases slightly. Filtering performance, however, becomes more dependent on the ability to obtain accurate motion vectors.

Figures 5–8 show several processed clinical frames of the image sequence, for $\lambda = 0.75$. It can be seen that the temporal filter does a better job over spatial filtering in terms of filtering out the quantum-mottle evident in the degraded images. This supports the numbers obtained from the I_{SNR} criterion.

3.6. RECURSIVE LINEAR TEMPORAL FILTERING

In this section, a finite tap LMMSE estimator is derived for the temporal filtering of image sequences corrupted by quantum-limited noise. This linear estimator is the recursive counterpart of the multiple input LLMMSE filter presented in the previous section. Recursive estimators are of considerable interest in applications such as those where real-time processing is crucial,[59] as in the case here.

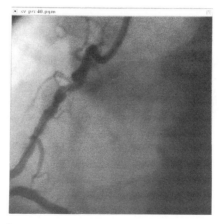

Figure 5. Original frame 40 for fluoro sequence.

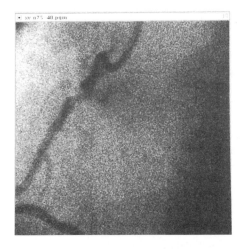

Figure 6. Degraded frame 40 at $\lambda = 0.75$.

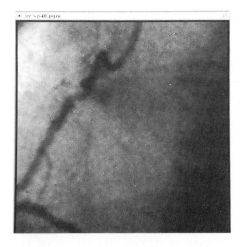

Figure 7. Spatially filtered frame 40.

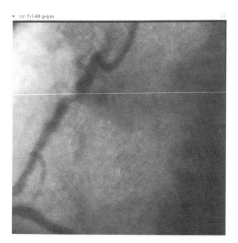

Figure 8. MC temporally filtered frame 40.

3.6.1. Recursive Filter Formulation

Consider, again, the LLMMSE filter in Equation (12). In this section, a temporally recursive sliding window multiple-input filter is developed to recover each frame of the degraded image sequence, whereby the filter operates on K motion-compensated frames (i.e., K causal taps) at a time.[12] Bringing back into the notation the temporal independent variable, p, the operation of this filter entails getting a filtered estimate at the p-th temporal position at each pixel according to

$$\hat{f}^{(p)}(\mathbf{r}) = \bar{f}^{(p)}(\mathbf{r}) + \begin{bmatrix} v^{(p)}_{fg^{MC}_{p-K+1}}(\mathbf{r}) \\ v^{(p)}_{fg^{MC}_{p-K+2}}(\mathbf{r}) \\ \vdots \\ v^{(p)}_{fg_p}(\mathbf{r}) \end{bmatrix}^{T}$$

$$\begin{bmatrix} v^{(p)}_{g^{MC}_{p-K+1}g^{MC}_{p-K+1}}(\mathbf{r}) & v^{(p)}_{g^{MC}_{p-K+1}g^{MC}_{p-K+2}}(\mathbf{r}) & \cdots & v^{(p)}_{g^{MC}_{p-K+1}g_p}(\mathbf{r}) \\ v^{(p)}_{g^{MC}_{p-K+2}g^{MC}_{p-K+1}}(\mathbf{r}) & v^{(p)}_{g^{MC}_{p-K+2}g^{MC}_{p-K+2}}(\mathbf{r}) & \cdots & v^{(p)}_{g^{MC}_{p-K+2}g_p}(\mathbf{r}) \\ & \vdots & & \\ v^{(p)}_{g_p g^{MC}_{p-K+1}}(\mathbf{r}) & v^{(p)}_{g_p g^{MC}_{p-K+2}}(\mathbf{r}) & \cdots & v^{(p)}_{g_p g_p}(\mathbf{r}) \end{bmatrix}^{-1}$$

$$
\cdot \begin{bmatrix} g_{p-K+1}^{MC}(\mathbf{r}) - \bar{g}_{p-K+1}^{MC}(\mathbf{r}) \\ g_{p-K+2}^{MC}(\mathbf{r}) - \bar{g}_{p-K+2}^{MC}(\mathbf{r}) \\ \vdots \\ g_p(\mathbf{r}) - \bar{g}_p(\mathbf{r}) \end{bmatrix}. \tag{17}
$$

The local statistics are estimated from the degraded data, with the p-th estimate of the local mean of $\mathbf{f}$ given by

$$
\bar{f}^{(p)}(\mathbf{r}) = \frac{1}{p S_W} \left[\sum_{i=1}^{p-1} \sum_{\mathbf{w} \in W} g_i^{MC}(\mathbf{r} + \mathbf{w}) + \sum_{\mathbf{w} \in W} g_p(\mathbf{r} + \mathbf{w}) \right], \tag{18}
$$

where W is a 2-D uniform moving average support window with S_W pixels, and the superscript MC represents the degraded frame motion-compensated to the current p-th working frame. Using the additive noise model in Equation (7), the local mean of each degraded frame in Equation (17) is equal to the local mean of $\mathbf{f}$ at time p; that is,

$$
\bar{g}_i^{MC}(\mathbf{r}) = \bar{f}^{(p)}(\mathbf{r}), \qquad \forall i = p - K + 1, \dots, p - 1, \tag{19}
$$

and

$$
\bar{g}_p(\mathbf{r}) = \bar{f}^{(p)}(\mathbf{r}). \tag{20}
$$

Although only K causal taps are considered in the filter, all of the past frames (i.e., $1, \dots, p$) are used to compute the first and second order moments, unlike the nonrecursive filter in Equation (12). This technique provides for a better estimate of these quantities as the number of samples increases, while simultaneously keeping the dimensionality of the problem constant by only considering K taps at a time.

It is straightforward to see, then, that the sample averages can be updated with the introduction of a new frame. Specifically, the updated local statistics can be written in a manner that allows for a recursive implementation. For example, the $(p + 1)$-th estimate of the local mean of $\mathbf{f}$ is given by

$$
\bar{f}^{(p+1)}(\mathbf{r}) = \frac{1}{(p+1) S_W} \left[\sum_{i=1}^{p} \sum_{\mathbf{w} \in W} g_i(\mathbf{r} - \mathbf{d}_{i,p+1}(\mathbf{r}) + \mathbf{w}) \right.
$$

$$
\left. + \sum_{\mathbf{w} \in W} g_{p+1}(\mathbf{r} + \mathbf{w}) \right]
$$

$$
= \frac{1}{p+1} \left[p \bar{f}^{(p)MC}(\mathbf{r}) + \frac{1}{S_W} \sum_{\mathbf{w} \in W} g_{p+1}(\mathbf{r} + \mathbf{w}) \right], \tag{21}
$$

where $\bar{f}^{(p)MC}(\mathbf{r})$ is the p-th estimate of $\bar{f}(\mathbf{r})$ motion-compensated to the $(p+1)$-th frame. The second step allows for the computation of this quantity without having to actually motion-compensate all of the past p frames to the current $(p+1)$-th frame at each step. Since

$$\bar{f}^{(p)MC}(\mathbf{r}) = \bar{f}^{(p)}(\mathbf{r} - \mathbf{d}_{p,p+1}(\mathbf{r})), \qquad (22)$$

this quantity may be found either by local sample averaging at each pixel of $\hat{f}^{(p)MC}$ using

$$\bar{f}^{(p)MC}(\mathbf{r}) = \frac{1}{S_W} \sum_{\mathbf{w} \in W} \hat{f}^{(p)MC}(\mathbf{r} + \mathbf{w}) \qquad (23)$$

or by treating the set of local means at each pixel as intensity values and projecting them forward to the $(p+1)$-th frame using the estimated DVF according to Equation (22). The sample averaging technique of Equation (23) gives slightly better results experimentally and was used instead. This may be attributed to the fact that the intensity values (or local means, here) need to be interpolated since the values of the DVF are non-integer.

The local mean, $\bar{f}^{(p)}$, is used to form a set of residual images[44] for use in the recursive filter. Essentially, this local mean is subtracted from the set of K motion-compensated observations resulting in a vector of zero-mean residuals. Let

$$
\begin{aligned}
y_i(\mathbf{r}) &= g_i^{MC}(\mathbf{r}) - \bar{g}_i^{MC}(\mathbf{r}) \\
&= g_i^{MC}(\mathbf{r}) - \bar{f}^{(p)}(\mathbf{r}), \qquad \forall i = p - K + 1, \ldots, p - 1,
\end{aligned}
\qquad (24)
$$

and

$$y_p(\mathbf{r}) = g_p(\mathbf{r}) - \bar{f}^{(p)}(\mathbf{r}), \qquad (25)$$

be the set of residual observations. Clearly, each $y_i(\mathbf{r})$ has zero-mean. In addition, let

$$x(\mathbf{r}) = f(\mathbf{r}) - \bar{f}(\mathbf{r}). \qquad (26)$$

Then Equation (17) can be rewritten as

$$\hat{x}^{(p)}(\mathbf{r}) = \begin{bmatrix} R^{(p)}_{xy^{MC}_{p-K+1}}(\mathbf{r}) \\ R^{(p)}_{xy^{MC}_{p-K+2}}(\mathbf{r}) \\ \vdots \\ R^{(p)}_{xy_p}(\mathbf{r}) \end{bmatrix}^{T}$$

$$\cdot \begin{bmatrix} R^{(p)}_{y^{MC}_{p-K+1}y^{MC}_{p-K+1}}(\mathbf{r}) & R^{(p)}_{y^{MC}_{p-K+1}y^{MC}_{p-K+2}}(\mathbf{r}) & \cdots & R^{(p)}_{y^{MC}_{p-K+1}y_p}(\mathbf{r}) \\ R^{(p)}_{y^{MC}_{p-K+2}y^{MC}_{p-K+1}}(\mathbf{r}) & R^{(p)}_{y^{MC}_{p-K+2}y^{MC}_{p-K+2}}(\mathbf{r}) & \cdots & R^{(p)}_{y^{MC}_{p-K+2}y_p}(\mathbf{r}) \\ & \vdots & & \\ R^{(p)}_{y_p y^{MC}_{p-K+1}}(\mathbf{r}) & R^{(p)}_{y_p y^{MC}_{p-K+2}}(\mathbf{r}) & \cdots & R^{(p)}_{y_p y_p}(\mathbf{r}) \end{bmatrix}^{-1}$$

$$\cdot \begin{bmatrix} y^{MC}_{p-K+1}(\mathbf{r}) \\ y^{MC}_{p-K+2}(\mathbf{r}) \\ \vdots \\ y_p(\mathbf{r}) \end{bmatrix}, \tag{27}$$

where the $(p+1)$-st sample cross-correlation, $R^{(p+1)}_{y_i y_j}(\mathbf{r})$, at pixel location $\mathbf{r}$, is equal to the sum of two terms: (a) the p-th sample cross-correlation, $R^{(p)MC}_{y_i y_j}(\mathbf{r})$, which is motion-compensated to the current frame and weighted by the number of previous samples and (b) the current sample, $y_{p+1}(\mathbf{r})$, cross-correlated to the previous sample at $(p+1)-\tau$ which is motion-compensated to the current frame. Specifically,

$$R^{(p+1)}_{y_i y_j}(\mathbf{r}) = \frac{1}{p+1}\left\{pR^{(p)MC}_{y_i y_j}(\mathbf{r}) + y^{MC}_{(p+1)-\tau}(\mathbf{r})y_{p+1}(\mathbf{r})\right\}, \tag{28}$$

$$\forall \tau = |i - j|.$$

Similarly, the cross-correlation between x and y_i, at pixel location $\mathbf{r}$, is given by

$$R^{(p+1)}_{xy_i}(\mathbf{r}) = \frac{1}{p+1}\left\{pR^{(p)MC}_{xy_i}(\mathbf{r}) + \hat{x}^{(p)MC}(\mathbf{r})y_{p+1}(\mathbf{r})\right\}. \tag{29}$$

The p-th estimate of the original image, $\hat{f}^{(p)}(\mathbf{r})$, can be obtained by solving Equation (27) for $\hat{x}^{(p)}(\mathbf{r})$ and adding the local mean $\bar{f}^{(p)}(\mathbf{r})$ back.

As shown below, the purpose of a recursive implementation is to provide a means of inverting the correlation matrix in Equation (27) in a recursive fashion to achieve computational efficiency. In recursively updating the inverse of the correlation matrix, however, the terms $R_{y_i y_j}^{(p)MC}(\mathbf{r})$ and $R_{xy_i}^{(p)MC}(\mathbf{r})$ in Equations (28) and (29) are not useful since they themselves cannot be computed recursively due to the need for motion compensation of all past estimates to the current frame. Therefore, instead of motion compensating all past correlation estimates, an optional exponential forgetting factor, μ, is introduced which weights the effect of past data with no motion-compensation on the sample average of the correlation terms. Thus, the recursive update of the correlation terms in Equations (28) and (29) becomes

$$R_{y_i y_j}^{(p+1)}(\mathbf{r}) \approx \frac{1}{p+1}\left\{ \mu p R_{y_i y_j}^{(p)}(\mathbf{r}) + y_{(p+1)-\tau}^{MC}(\mathbf{r})y_{(p+1)}(\mathbf{r})\right\},$$

$$\forall \tau = |i - j|,$$

(30)

and

$$R_{xy_i}^{(p+1)}(\mathbf{r}) \approx \frac{1}{p+1}\left\{ \mu p R_{xy_i}^{(p)}(\mathbf{r}) + \hat{x}^{(p)MC}(\mathbf{r})y_{(p+1)}(\mathbf{r})\right\}. \quad (31)$$

Note that the forgetting factor is not used in the recursive updating of the local mean since the motion-compensated local mean can be computed at each step using Equation (23).

Because the update of local statistics can be seen to be a straightforward process, the incorporation of new data in the filter can be done in a recursive fashion as well, enabling a less computationally intensive procedure in an intuitive manner. Furthermore, information about past estimates can be used to improve upon future estimates. In developing a recursive filter, the expression in Equation (27) may be rewritten as

$$\hat{x}^{(p)}(\mathbf{r}) = \phi^T(p)\Phi^{-1}(p)\begin{bmatrix} y_{p-K+1}^{MC}(\mathbf{r}) \\ y_{p-K+2}^{MC}(\mathbf{r}) \\ \vdots \\ y_p(\mathbf{r}) \end{bmatrix}$$

$$= \begin{bmatrix} \beta_{p-K+1}(\mathbf{r}) \\ \vdots \\ \beta_p(\mathbf{r}) \end{bmatrix}^T \begin{bmatrix} y_{p-K+1}^{MC}(\mathbf{r}) \\ y_{p-K+2}^{MC}(\mathbf{r}) \\ \vdots \\ y_p(\mathbf{r}) \end{bmatrix}$$

$$= \gamma^T(p) \begin{bmatrix} y_{p-K+1}^{MC}(\mathbf{r}) \\ y_{p-K+2}^{MC}(\mathbf{r}) \\ \vdots \\ y_p(\mathbf{r}) \end{bmatrix}, \qquad (32)$$

where $\gamma(p)$ is the vector of optimal coefficients to be determined, $\Phi^{-1}(p)$ is the inverse of the correlation matrix to be inverted and $\phi(p)$ is the correlation vector, all at time p. The correlation matrix, which is symmetric, is given by

$$\Phi(p) = \begin{bmatrix} R_{y_{p-K+1}^{MC}y_{p-K+1}^{MC}}^{(p)}(\mathbf{r}) & R_{y_{p-K+1}^{MC}y_{p-K+2}^{MC}}^{(p)}(\mathbf{r}) & \cdots & R_{y_{p-K+1}^{MC}y_p}^{(p)}(\mathbf{r}) \\ R_{y_{p-K+2}^{MC}y_{p-K+1}^{MC}}^{(p)}(\mathbf{r}) & R_{y_{p-K+2}^{MC}y_{p-K+2}^{MC}}^{(p)}(\mathbf{r}) & \cdots & R_{y_{p-K+2}^{MC}y_p}^{(p)}(\mathbf{r}) \\ & \vdots & & \\ R_{y_p y_{p-K+1}^{MC}}^{(p)}(\mathbf{r}) & R_{y_p y_{p-K+2}^{MC}}^{(p)}(\mathbf{r}) & \cdots & R_{y_p y_p}^{(p)}(\mathbf{r}) \end{bmatrix} \qquad (33)$$

and the correlation vector is given by

$$\phi(p) = \begin{bmatrix} R_{xy_{p-K+1}^{MC}}^{(p)}(\mathbf{r}) \\ R_{xy_{p-K+2}^{MC}}^{(p)}(\mathbf{r}) \\ \vdots \\ R_{xy_p}^{(p)}(\mathbf{r}) \end{bmatrix}. \qquad (34)$$

Let $\Phi(p+1)$ be the correlation matrix after the introduction of the $(p+1)$-st sample from the new frame. Using Equation (30), the updated covariance matrix can be written as

$$\Phi(p+1) = \mu \left(\frac{p}{p+1} \right) \Phi(p) + \frac{1}{p+1} u_{p+1}(\mathbf{r}) u_{p+1}(\mathbf{r})^T, \qquad (35)$$

where

$$u_{p+1}(\mathbf{r}) = \begin{bmatrix} y_{p-K+2}^{MC}(\mathbf{r}) \\ \vdots \\ y_{p+1}(\mathbf{r}) \end{bmatrix}. \tag{36}$$

Essentially, the expression in Equation (35) represents the renormalization of the covariance matrix after the addition of a new observation. Similarly, using Equation (31), the updated cross-correlation vector can be written as

$$\phi(p+1) = \mu\left(\frac{p}{p+1}\right)\phi(p) + \frac{1}{p+1}\hat{x}^{(p)}(\mathbf{r} - \hat{\mathbf{d}}_{p,p+1}(\mathbf{r}))u_{p+1}(\mathbf{r}). \tag{37}$$

Making use of the matrix inversion lemma,[36]

$$\left[A^{-1} + B^T C^{-1} B\right]^{-1} = A - AB^T\left[BAB^T + C\right]^{-1}BA, \tag{38}$$

for the matrices A, B, and C, it can be shown that the inverse of $\Phi(p+1)$ is given by

$$\Phi^{-1}(p+1) = \frac{1}{\mu}\left(\frac{p+1}{p}\right)\Phi^{-1}(p)$$
$$- \frac{\frac{1}{\mu^2}\left(\frac{p+1}{p}\right)^2\Phi^{-1}(p)u_{p+1}(\mathbf{r})u_{p+1}^T(\mathbf{r})\Phi^{-1}(p)}{(p+1) + \frac{1}{\mu}\left(\frac{p+1}{p}\right)u_{p+1}^T(\mathbf{r})\Phi^{-1}(p)u_{p+1}(\mathbf{r})}. \tag{39}$$

The updated unknown coefficient vector can then be given by

$$\gamma(p+1) = \Phi^{-1}(p+1)\phi(p+1). \tag{40}$$

Consequently, the estimate of the next frame given the new observation becomes

$$\hat{f}^{(p+1)}(\mathbf{r}) = \bar{f}^{(p+1)}(\mathbf{r}) + \gamma^T(p+1)u_{p+1}(\mathbf{r}), \tag{41}$$

where the local mean was added back to the estimate, $\hat{x}^{(p+1)}$. A block diagram of the recursive filter described above is shown in Figure 9.

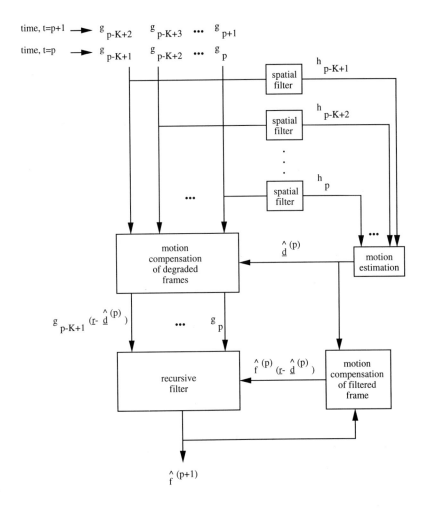

Figure 9. Block diagram of motion-compensated recursive temporal filter.

3.6.2. Initialization and Implementation Details

The recursive updating of the correlation matrix, $\Phi(p)$, in Equation (35) and the cross-correlation vector, $\phi(p)$, in Equation (37) needs to be initialized for the first step. Since the filter is causal and possesses K taps, the values of $\Phi(K)$ and $\phi(K)$ or their inverses must be pre-specified before the recursion can begin. For this initialization stage, a more robust means of computing each element's local statistics is provided. Specifically, the cross-correlation terms, $R_{y_i y_j}(\mathbf{r})$, are found by using the fact that

$$\mathbf{R}_{y_i y_j} = \mathbf{C}_{g_i g_j} = E\{(\mathbf{g}_i - E\{\mathbf{g}_i\})(\mathbf{g}_j - E\{\mathbf{g}_j\})\}$$

$$= E\{(\mathbf{f} + \mathbf{n}_i - E\{\mathbf{f}\})(\mathbf{f} + \mathbf{n}_j - E\{\mathbf{f}\})\}$$

$$= \mathbf{C}_f, \tag{42}$$

where $\mathbf{y}_i$ is the residual observed image and $\mathbf{R}_{y_i y_j}$ is the cross-correlation matrix between $\mathbf{y}_i$ and $\mathbf{y}_j$. Similarly, the cross-covariance matrices, $\mathbf{R}_{xy_i}$, can be rewritten as

$$\mathbf{R}_{xy_i} = \mathbf{C}_{fg_i} = E\{(\mathbf{f} - E\{\mathbf{f}\})(\mathbf{g}_i - E\{\mathbf{g}_i\})\}$$

$$= E\{(\mathbf{f} - E\{\mathbf{f}\})(\mathbf{f} + \mathbf{n}_i - E\{\mathbf{f}\})\}$$

$$= \mathbf{C}_f. \tag{43}$$

The covariance matrices $\mathbf{C}_f$ in Equations (42) and (43) are given by

$$\mathbf{C}_f = \sigma_f^2(\mathbf{r})\mathbf{I}, \tag{44}$$

where the local mean of $f(\mathbf{r})$ is approximated again using Equation (18) and $p = K$. The local variance of $f(\mathbf{r})$ is given instead by

$$\sigma_f^2(\mathbf{r}) = \frac{1}{K} \sum_{k=1}^{K} \left[\sigma_{g_k}^2(\mathbf{r}) - \frac{1}{\lambda} \bar{f}(\mathbf{r}) \right], \tag{45}$$

where the Poisson noise statistics derived in Section 3.3 were used for the computation of the noise variance.

Substituting Equations (42), (43), and (44) into Equation (32), the initial correlation matrix, $\Phi(K)$, for the first K frames, becomes

$$\Phi(K) = \begin{bmatrix} \sigma_{g_1^{MC}}^2(\mathbf{r}) & \sigma_f^2(\mathbf{r}) & \cdots & \sigma_f^2(\mathbf{r}) \\ \sigma_f^2(\mathbf{r}) & \sigma_{g_2^{MC}}^2(\mathbf{r}) & \cdots & \sigma_f^2(\mathbf{r}) \\ & & \ddots & \\ \sigma_f^2(\mathbf{r}) & \sigma_f^2(\mathbf{r}) & \cdots & \sigma_{g_K}^2(\mathbf{r}) \end{bmatrix}. \tag{46}$$

The inverse of $\Phi(K)$ (which can be accomplished using singular value decomposition methods) is assumed to exist and serves as an initial point for the recursion process. Similarly, the initial cross-covariance vector, $\phi(K)$, for the first K frames, is given by

$$\phi(K) = \begin{bmatrix} \sigma_f^2(\mathbf{r}) \\ \sigma_f^2(\mathbf{r}) \\ \vdots \\ \sigma_f^2(\mathbf{r}) \end{bmatrix}. \tag{47}$$

These two quantities, $\Phi(K)$ and $\phi(K)$, may be used to obtain an initial estimate of the image, $\hat{f}^{(K)}$, given K degraded frames using Equations (40) and (41).

It should be noted that the recursive filter has its own shortcomings due to the dynamic behavior of the sequence. If the displacement vector estimates are not accurate for a particular set of frames, errors will accumulate in subsequent filtered frames. Usually, this may be remedied by setting the forgetting factor, μ, to a value below unity. However, this introduces bias effects that can dramatically alter the filter performance. For this reason, the simulation experiments here all utilized a forgetting factor close to unity, i.e., $\mu = 0.997$. Another alternative may be to reinitialize the recursive filter after some time interval.

As noted earlier, the recursion process builds up the temporal support window used to estimate the local statistics with the addition of each new sample. The size of the spatial analysis window can thus be decreased at the expense of the gradual increase in temporal support. This reduces the computational intensity as there will be fewer elements to consider at each pixel as well as reducing the possibility of including a discontinuity in the window. Consequently, a 7×7 spatial analysis window is used for the first K frames and the size of the window is decreased to a 3×3 window for the next and subsequent frames.

3.6.3. Experimental Results

The temporally recursive filter proposed in the previous section was applied to 10 frames of a noisy clinical X-ray image sequence with inherent quantum noise. Here, a block matching algorithm is used to obtain the DVF with no spatial filtering preprocessing stage, since the noise is low enough for the algorithm to yield good vector fields. The value of λ can be estimated from a homogeneous region of the image using sample averaging. Specifically, it is known from Equation (4) that

$$\sigma_n^2(\mathbf{r}) = \frac{1}{\lambda} E\{f(\mathbf{r})\}. \tag{48}$$

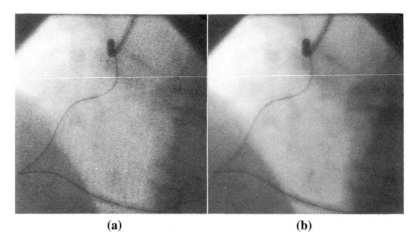

(a)   **(b)**

Figure 10. (a) Frame 13 of clinical sequence (b) Recursively temporally filtered frame 13.

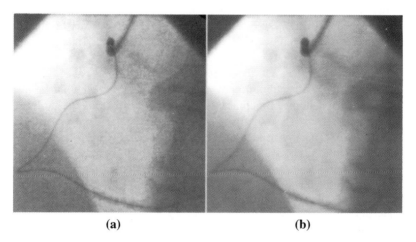

(a)   **(b)**

Figure 11. (a) Frame 14 of clinical sequence (b) Recursively temporally filtered frame 14.

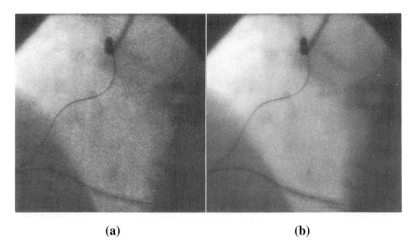

(a)   **(b)**

Figure 12. (a) Frame 15 of clinical sequence (b) Recursively temporally filtered frame 15.

Using sample averaging to compute both $E\{f(\mathbf{r})\}$ and $\sigma_{n_g}^2(\mathbf{r})$ within the homogeneous region, λ can be estimated using this relation. For the clinical sequence, it is observed from Figures 10(a), 11(a), and 12(a), that the noise level is less (estimated $\lambda \approx 10$) than that simulated in the clinical sequence (c.f. Figure 6). This is due to the limitation of the X-ray generator used in this and most other fluoroscopy units. In the experiments, this is the lowest selectable dosage for clinical use without reconfiguring the hardware parameters. Because this noise is not simulated, the same I_{SNR} criterion in Equation (16) cannot be used to assess the performance of the filter, since an "original frame" is not available for comparison. Instead, three consecutive frames of the sequence are shown in Figures 10–12 along with their recursive temporally filtered versions for comparison.

Though, individually, the unprocessed frames themselves do not look noisy enough to warrant processing, viewing them at video rate introduces enough flicker from frame to frame to be objectionable to radiologists 23. The processed sequence viewed at the same video rate does not have this problem because of the increased smoothness afforded by the recursive filter.

From the experiments, it can be seen that the proposed algorithm can handle various levels of quantum noise — from moderate to severe. Although the use of lower X-ray dosage levels with current fluoroscopy units is not done because of the quantum noise that arises, the simulations here show that these lower levels, more preferable for reasons of safety, can be implemented provided an algorithm for postprocessing, such as the one proposed here, is available. In addition, the recursive temporal filter is also applicable to quantum-limited images where the light is naturally low due to the imaging conditions such as astronomical imaging, low-light level remote sensing and surveillance videos.

3.7. LINEAR QUADRATIC TEMPORAL FILTERING

The techniques introduced for temporal filtering of image sequences so far in Sections 3.5 and 3.6 represent locally optimal linear estimates of the unknown signal. Specifically, the form of the estimator at each pixel was constrained to be a linear function of the observed data. This provided a tractable solution with reasonable filter performance over the linear spatial filter. However, with the MMSE criterion, the ultimate solution in Equation (1) is in finding the conditional mean, which is, in general, a nonlinear function of the observed data for the quantum-limited noise case. Though the use of linear filters may be sufficient, nonlinear filters can provide additional improvement for non Gaussian processes. This is especially true for the Poisson noise case because it is known to have information in the higher order moments.

In this section, the means through which this performance improvement can be obtained is examined by looking at a class of nonlinear systems describable by a Volterra expansion.[68] Specifically, a set of linear-quadratic filters is derived using higher order statistics for suppressing the quantum noise without the need to know the exact pdf governing the noise samples.

Using the additive-signal model in Equation (1), a suboptimal nonlinear estimator can be derived based on the use of higher-order moments. Such an estimator is more reasonable since the degradation, mathematically modeled as a Poisson-distributed noise source, cannot be uniquely characterized by the 1st and 2nd order moments alone. Additional information may be gained from knowledge or estimation of higher order moments. Based on these moments, a linear-quadratic estimator is derived, where the probability distribution of the noise term is approximated by a distribution with truncated moments.

The general form of the p-th order one-dimensional discrete-time FIR Volterra filter (VF) is a nonlinear structure whose input-output relationship can be given by [69]

$$\hat{f} = f_0 + \sum_{m=1}^{p} \sum_{\{i_n^m\}} h_m \left[i_1^m, i_2^m, \dots, i_m^m \right] g \left[i_1^m \right] g \left[i_2^m \right] \cdots g \left[i_m^m \right],$$

$$1 \le i_n^m \le N,$$

(49)

where $h_m \left[i_1^m, i_2^m, \ldots, i_m^m \right]$ denotes the m-dimensional filter weight sequence, and g and f are the filter's input and output. Essentially, this is a filter based on an exhaustive correlation between pixels in the region of support. In this chapter, only 2nd-order VFs ($p = 2$), corresponding to a linear-quadratic (LQ) filter[68], are considered. Eykhoff has an explicit form for the one-dimensional p-th order Volterra filter based on a minimum MSE criterion.[24]

This form written for the 2nd-order two-dimensional Volterra filter is given by

$$\hat{f}(\mathbf{r}) = f_0 + \sum_{\mathbf{x} \in \Re} \alpha(\mathbf{x}) g(\mathbf{r} + \mathbf{x}) + \sum_{\mathbf{x} \in \Re} \sum_{\mathbf{y} \in \Re} \beta(\mathbf{x}, \mathbf{y}) g(\mathbf{r} + \mathbf{x}) g(\mathbf{r} + \mathbf{y}), \quad (50)$$

where $\alpha(\mathbf{x})$ and $\beta(\mathbf{x}, \mathbf{y})$ are the Volterra filter weights, and $\Re$ is the support of the filter. Koh and Powers have shown that the absence of the zeroth-order term, f_0, might cause the filter output to become biased.[52] Assuming that the observation and the original signal are zero-mean, the Volterra filter weights are found here through a minimization of the mean square error. This assumption is not overly restrictive and is made here only for convenience of notation, since zero-mean residuals can be formed from the observations (e.g., by subtracting out the local mean and adding it back after filtering). It can be shown [52] that the zeroth-order term is given by

$$f_0 = -\sum_{\mathbf{x} \in \Re} \sum_{\mathbf{y} \in \Re} \beta(\mathbf{x}, \mathbf{y}) R_g(\mathbf{x}, \mathbf{y}) \quad (51)$$

for the two-dimensional 2nd-order VF.

In general, the inversion of a $M(M + 3)/2$ by $M(M + 3)/2$ matrix is necessary for the 2nd order Volterra filter with a support of M pixels.[52] Similarly, a VF of order p suffers the additional problem of higher-order statistics (HOS) estimation as it requires knowledge of $2p$ autocorrelation functions and p cross-correlation functions.[52] So a filter of order $p > 2$ becomes increasingly less reliable if the higher order moments can only be derived from the degraded samples. For this reason, only 2nd order VF's are considered corresponding to LQ filters.

3.7.1. Spatial Filtering

Consider the LQ form of the following estimator:

$$\hat{f}(\mathbf{r}) = f_0 + \alpha g(\mathbf{r}) + \beta g^2(\mathbf{r}) \quad (52)$$

where $g(\mathbf{r})$ is the observation at the $\mathbf{r}$-th pixel location. It is desired to find the optimal minimum mean square error estimate of $f(\mathbf{r})$, the true intensity signal, by finding the optimal coefficients α, β, and f_0. The mean square error of the VF is orthogonal not only to the observation, but also to all possible products of the observation. Therefore, minimizing the mean square prediction error is equivalent to solving the following system of equations:

$$\begin{bmatrix} R_{gg} & R_{ggg} \\ R_{ggg} & R_{gggg} - R_{gg}^2 \end{bmatrix} \begin{bmatrix} \alpha \\ \beta \end{bmatrix} = \begin{bmatrix} R_{fg} \\ R_{fgg} \end{bmatrix} \tag{53}$$

and

$$f_0 = -\beta(\mathbf{r})E\{g^2(\mathbf{r})\}, \tag{54}$$

where

$$R_{gg} = E\{g(\mathbf{r})g(\mathbf{r})\}$$

$$R_{ggg} = E\{g(\mathbf{r})g(\mathbf{r})g(\mathbf{r})\}$$

$$R_{gggg} = E\{g(\mathbf{r})g(\mathbf{r})g(\mathbf{r})g(\mathbf{r})\}. \tag{55}$$

These correlations are estimated using sample moments obtained from the degraded image(s). The cross-correlations, R_{fg} and R_{fgg}, are equal to (see Appendix)

$$R_{fg} = E\{f^2(\mathbf{r})\} \tag{56}$$

and

$$R_{fgg} = \frac{1}{\lambda}E\{f^2(\mathbf{r})\} + E\{f^3(\mathbf{r})\}$$

$$= E\{g^3(\mathbf{r})\} - \frac{1}{\lambda^2}E\{f(\mathbf{r})\} - \frac{2}{\lambda}E\{f^2(\mathbf{r})\}. \tag{57}$$

3.7.2. Multichannel Filtering

In this section, the formulation of the linear quadratic spatial filter is extended to the multichannel case for the arbitrary case when K multiple frames of the same scene are available. The K-frame LQ multichannel filter is given by Equation (50) modified here to show the increased support

$$\hat{f}(\mathbf{r}) = f_0 + \sum_{k=1}^{K} \alpha(k) g_k(\mathbf{r}) + \sum_{k=1}^{K} \sum_{l=1}^{K} \beta(k,l) g_k(\mathbf{r}) g_l(\mathbf{r}). \qquad (58)$$

Let the set of the K observations in the support be stacked into a vector $\mathbf{g}$ where

$$\mathbf{g} = [g_1(\mathbf{r}), g_2(\mathbf{r}), \dots, g_K(\mathbf{r})]^T \qquad (59)$$

with covariance matrix

$$\mathbf{C} = E\{\mathbf{g}\mathbf{g}^T\}. \qquad (60)$$

Furthermore, let $\mathbf{h}$ be the vector of unknown coefficients for the linear terms and $\mathbf{H}$ the matrix of unknown coefficients for the quadratic terms

$$\mathbf{h} = \begin{bmatrix} \alpha(1) \\ \alpha(2) \\ \vdots \\ \alpha(K) \end{bmatrix}, \quad \mathbf{H} = \begin{bmatrix} \beta(1,1) & \beta(1,2) & \cdots & \beta(1,K) \\ \beta(2,1) & \beta(2,2) & \cdots & \beta(2,K) \\ & & \vdots & \\ \beta(K,1) & \beta(K,2) & \cdots & \beta(K,K) \end{bmatrix}. \qquad (61)$$

Then the K-frame LQ multichannel filter can be written in the following compact form[68]

$$\hat{f}(\mathbf{r}) = f_0 + \mathbf{h}^T \mathbf{g} + \mathbf{g}^T \mathbf{H} \mathbf{g} \qquad (62)$$

where

$$f_0 = -\mathrm{Tr}(\mathbf{CH}) \qquad (63)$$

for the estimator to have zero bias. The optimal pair, $[\mathbf{h_o}, \mathbf{H_o}]$, can be found through a minimization of the mean square error

$$[\mathbf{h_o}, \mathbf{H_o}] \leftarrow \min_{[\mathbf{h}, \mathbf{H}]} E\left\{ \left[f(\mathbf{r}) - \hat{f}(\mathbf{r}) \right]^2 \right\}. \qquad (64)$$

To provide some insight into the performance and computational complexity of this filter, it is useful to examine the 2-frame case. This LQ estimator is given by

$$\hat{f}(\mathbf{r}) = f_0 + \alpha_1 g_1(\mathbf{r}) + \alpha_2 g_2(\mathbf{r}) + \beta_1 g_1^2(\mathbf{r}) + \beta_2 g_1(\mathbf{r}) g_2(\mathbf{r}) + \beta_3 g_2^2(\mathbf{r}), \quad (65)$$

where $f(\mathbf{r})$ is the true signal intensity at the $\mathbf{r}$-th pixel location, $g_1(\mathbf{r})$ and $g_2(\mathbf{r})$ are the two observations of the same scene, and $\alpha_1 \overset{\text{def}}{=} \alpha(1), \alpha_2 \overset{\text{def}}{=} \alpha(2)$, $\beta_1 \overset{\text{def}}{=} \beta(1, 1)$, and $\beta_3 \overset{\text{def}}{=} \beta(2, 2)$. Because of certain symmetries in the lag vectors of the moments[28], $\beta(1, 2) = \beta(2, 1)$; consequently,

$$\beta_2 \overset{\text{def}}{=} \frac{1}{2}[\beta(1, 2) + \beta(2, 1)] = \beta(1, 2). \qquad (66)$$

Minimizing the mean square prediction error to find the optimal coefficients is equivalent to solving the following system of equations

$$
\begin{bmatrix}
R_{g_1^2} & R_{g_1 g_2} & R_{g_1^3} & R_{g_1^2 g_2} & R_{g_2^2 g_1} \\
R_{g_1 g_2} & R_{g_2^2} & R_{g_1^2 g_2} & R_{g_1 g_2^2} & R_{g_2^3} \\
R_{g_1^3} & R_{g_2 g_1^2} & R_{g_1^4} - R_{g_1^2} & R_{g_1^3 g_2} - R_{g_1} R_{g_1 g_2} & R_{g_1^2 g_2^2} - R_{g_1} R_{g_2} \\
R_{g_2 g_1^2} & R_{g_2^2 g_1} & R_{g_1^3 g_2} - R_{g_1 g_2} R_{g_1} & R_{g_1^2 g_2^2} - R_{g_1 g_2}^2 & R_{g_1 g_2^3} - R_{g_1 g_2} R_{g_2} \\
R_{g_1 g_2^2} & R_{g_2^3} & R_{g_1^2 g_2^2} - R_{g_2} R_{g_1} & R_{g_1 g_2^3} - R_{g_2} R_{g_1 g_2} & R_{g_2^4} - R_{g_2^2}
\end{bmatrix}
$$

$$
\begin{bmatrix}
\alpha_1 \\
\alpha_2 \\
\beta_1 \\
\beta_2 \\
\beta_3
\end{bmatrix}
=
\begin{bmatrix}
R_{f g_1} \\
R_{f g_2} \\
R_{f g_1 g_1} \\
R_{f g_1 g_2} \\
R_{f g_2 g_2}
\end{bmatrix}
\qquad (67)
$$

and

$$f_0 = -\beta_1 E\{g_1^2(\mathbf{r})\} - \beta_2 E\{g_1(\mathbf{r})g_2(\mathbf{r})\} - \beta_3 E\{g_2^2(\mathbf{r})\}. \qquad (68)$$

The solution to this set of equations entails the inverse of a (5×5) matrix at each pixel, which is significantly more computationally intense than solving Equation (12) where only a (2×2) matrix needs to be inverted, for $K = 2$.

3.7.3. Discussion

Some preliminary work with this nonlinear filter has been done recently using nonclinical multichannel images simulated with Poisson noise.[17] Multichannel images can result from compensation for the motion of the frames in a dynamic image sequence as previously discussed in Section 3.4.1. In that study, it was found that the performance of the LQ filter on quantum mottled images varied depending on the type of images encountered. Specifically, improvement ranged from marginal for images with very little high frequency content to significant for images with a broader range of frequencies. This seemed to be consistent with Garth and Bresler's[32] work, where they found that higher order detection in narrowband processes to actually be inferior to linear detection.

Additional work is warranted in this area for clinical image sequences containing quantum-limited noise. For example, in the application of the temporal linear-quadratic filter to dynamic image sequences, it was observed that this filter's ability to reduce the mean square error was more susceptible to errors in motion estimation and compensation than the linear filter. A more accurate displacement field estimation algorithm may be necessary so that the estimation of the local statistics does not become skewed by registration artifacts. One possible solution is presented in the next section.

3.8. DISPLACEMENT FIELD ESTIMATION IN QUANTUM-LIMITED NOISE

In this section, an algorithm for the estimation of the DVF under the quantum-limited conditions is described. This method is different from the motion estimation methods discussed earlier in that it takes into account the underlying physical processes through which the image frames are acquired. Preliminary work using this method in phantoms and videoconferencing sequences simulated with quantum mottle show significant improvement in terms of both motion estimation and compensation.[16] It is anticipated that this method may be useful for low dose clinical angiography as well.

As mentioned earlier, there has been little work done on the displacement field estimation problem under quantum-limited noise conditions. Some work has been done, however, on the related one-dimensional counterpart of displacement field estimation; that is, the problem of time delay estimation under quantum-limited conditions. For example, Hero addresses the problem of time shift estimation in optical communications for both the Poisson-limited regime[38] and the mixed Poisson-Gaussian regime[39] from filtered Poisson point processes, or in the presence of shot noise. Antoniadis and Hero[3] implement an Expectation Maximization (EM)-type estimator[19] for the latter case in which the complete data consisted of the observation supplemented by the set of arrival times of each photoevent. Slocumb and Snyder[73] also use an EM algorithm in the closely related application of quantum-limited optical position sensing. In their paper, the spatial and temporal location of each photoevent occurring in the plane was assumed to be available for observation. For both of these applications, a localization of each photoevent is assumed to be feasible whether it is precisely known or is randomly translated. This scenario is not possible for the clinical angiography application since the imaging system cannot demarcate each of these events due to a finite pixel dimension and a finite integration time. Thus, the observed data in here is referred to as *histogram data* as opposed to *count-record data*.[75]

In count-record data applications,[40,73,74] the location of each photon detection is known subject to a random translation. In addition, the time of each detection is also known. Because the time-space location of each event is available, count-record data contains more information about the observed data than would histogram data, where only the number of events in each finite partition (i.e., pixel) of the detector space is known.

Based on this type of histogram data, an iterative Maximum Likelihood (ML) approach is described which uses a block component search algorithm[60] for the displacement field estimation problem without incorporating any knowledge of the photoevent locations. It will be shown in Section 3.8.1 that the difficulty in the evaluation of the log-likelihood function does not permit a tractable solution for the displacement field estimator when only the histogram data is available and not the count-record data. In light of this difficulty, the block component search algorithm is used for a joint estimation of the signal and the displacement.

3.8.1. Problem Formulation

Let $\mathbf{N_1}(A) = \chi(A, t_T) - \chi(A, t_0)$ and $\mathbf{N_2}(A) = \chi(A, t_{2T}) - \chi(A, t_T)$ be two-dimensional (2D) inhomogeneous Poisson counting processes observed in the intervals $[t_0, t_T)$ and $[t_T, t_{2T})$ respectively, and in the image plane $A \subset \mathcal{R}^2$. The counts correspond to the number of photons observed at the plane of the detector, A, in an imaging system. The point process, χ, is a doubly stochastic Poisson point process[20,75] with the spatially and temporally varying discrete intensity function,

$$\Lambda(\mathbf{r}, t, \mathbf{f}(\mathbf{r}, t)) = \sum_k \Lambda(\mathbf{r}, t_{kT}, \mathbf{f}(\mathbf{r}, t_{kT}))\delta(t - t_{kT}),$$

which governs the rate at which photons arrive and the number of photons observed. In other words, the conditional probability density function (pdf) has the form

$$p(\chi(A,t) = n|\mathbf{f}) = \frac{1}{n!} \left(\int_{[t_0,t) \times A} \Lambda(\mathbf{r}, \tau, \mathbf{f}(\mathbf{r}, \tau)) d\mathbf{r} d\tau \right)^n$$

$$\cdot \exp \left(- \int_{[t_0,t) \times A} \Lambda(\mathbf{r}, \tau, \mathbf{f}(\mathbf{r}, \tau)) d\mathbf{r} d\tau \right).$$

This intensity function, or rate, of the Poisson process is, in turn, governed by a random informational process, $\mathbf{f}(\mathbf{r}, t)$, that is assumed in to be linearly translating from $t_{(k-1)T}$ to t_{kT}:

$$\mathbf{f}(\mathbf{r}, t_{(k-1)T}) = \mathbf{f}(\mathbf{r} + \mathbf{d}(\mathbf{r}), t_{kT}), \qquad \forall k \in \mathcal{N} \qquad (69)$$

where $\mathbf{d}(\mathbf{r}) = \begin{bmatrix} d_x & d_y \end{bmatrix}^T$, assumed here to be unknown but nonrandom, is the displacement vector associated with a pixel at spatial location $\mathbf{r} = [x \ y]^T$ in the image. It will be shown later that the proposed algorithm results in a block matching algorithm with a nonlinear term to be maximized. It is assumed, as in block matching, that the vectors $\mathbf{d}(\mathbf{r})$ are constant within each block. Furthermore, the intensity function is assumed to be equal to the informational process, scaled by a proportionality factor, λ, which relates the displayed image intensity to the assumed number of photon counts present as shown in Figure 1,

$$\Lambda(\mathbf{r}, t_0, \mathbf{f}(\mathbf{r}, t_0)) = \lambda \mathbf{f}(\mathbf{r}, t_0) = \lambda \mathbf{f}(\mathbf{r} + \mathbf{d}(\mathbf{r}))$$

$$\Lambda(\mathbf{r}, t_1, \mathbf{f}(\mathbf{r}, t_1)) = \lambda \mathbf{f}(\mathbf{r}, t_1) = \lambda \mathbf{f}(\mathbf{r}),$$

where the time dependency has been removed in lieu of the characterization of the motion between two consecutive frames by the DVF alone. This is reasonable for sequences containing linear motion and no occlusions. In addition, the commonly made assumption that the image intensity is constant along the motion trajectory is made. The displacement vector field, $\mathbf{d}$, is denoted as the *set* of all displacement vectors, $\mathbf{d}(\mathbf{r})$ for $\mathbf{r} \in A$. The two Poisson counting processes represent two degraded image frames when the collected counts are appropriately mapped to intensity levels. These two image frames become perfectly registered when the condition in Equation (69) is satisfied $\forall \mathbf{r} \in A$.

Note that photoevents may occur in between the times $t_{(k-1)T}$ and t_{kT}, but again, the imaging system cannot demarcate each of these events. Conditioned on this informational process, $\mathbf{N_1}(A)$ and $\mathbf{N_2}(A)$ are conditional Poisson point processes for a given realization of the intensity function. Specifically,

$$p(\mathbf{N_1}|\mathbf{f}) = \prod_{\mathbf{r} \in A} p(\mathbf{N_1}(\mathbf{r}) = n_r | \mathbf{f}(\mathbf{r}))$$

$$= \prod_{\mathbf{r} \in A} [\lambda \mathbf{f}(\mathbf{r} + \mathbf{d}(\mathbf{r}))]^{n_r} \cdot \exp\{-\lambda \mathbf{f}(\mathbf{r} + \mathbf{d}(\mathbf{r}))\} / n_r! \tag{70}$$

and

$$p(\mathbf{N_2}|\mathbf{f}) = \prod_{\mathbf{r} \in A} p(\mathbf{N_2}(\mathbf{r}) = m_r | \mathbf{f}(\mathbf{r}))$$

$$= \prod_{\mathbf{r} \in A} [\lambda \mathbf{f}(\mathbf{r})]^{m_r} \exp\{-\lambda \mathbf{f}(\mathbf{r})\} / m_r! \tag{71}$$

where n_r and m_r are the observed counts at pixel location $\mathbf{r}$ in frames 1 and 2, respectively. The above assumption that the counting processes are statistically independent when conditioned on the informational process is justified for the low light-level situation.[56] Various image models may be used to characterize the informational process, $\mathbf{f}$. Again, as in the previous sections, $\mathbf{f}$ is assumed to be a multivariate Gaussian with a nonstationary mean, μ_f, and a nonstationary diagonal covariance matrix, Σ_f.[54]

The problem of displacement field estimation under quantum-limited conditions can be formulated using conventional Fisher maximum-likelihood techniques.[10] Specifically, it is desired to estimate the unknown nonrandom field, $\mathbf{d}$, from the two observed counting processes $\mathbf{N}_1$ and $\mathbf{N}_2$, or the observed degraded images, $\mathbf{g}_1$ and $\mathbf{g}_2$. Using the conditional density function for $\mathbf{g}_i(\mathbf{r})$ in Equation (3), the two conditional Poisson counting processes in Equations (70) and (71) may be rewritten as given by

$$p(\mathbf{g_1}|\mathbf{f}) = \prod_{\mathbf{r} \in A} \lambda \left[\lambda \mathbf{f}(\mathbf{r} + \mathbf{d}(\mathbf{r}))\right]^{\lambda \mathbf{g_1}(r)}$$

$$\exp\{-\lambda \mathbf{f}(\mathbf{r} + \mathbf{d}(\mathbf{r}))\} / \left[\lambda \mathbf{g_1}(\mathbf{r})\right]! \tag{72}$$

and

$$p(\mathbf{g_2}|\mathbf{f}) = \prod_{\mathbf{r} \in A} \lambda \left[\lambda \mathbf{f}(\mathbf{r})\right]^{\lambda \mathbf{g_2}(r)} \exp\{-\lambda \mathbf{f}(\mathbf{r})\} / \left[\lambda \mathbf{g_2}(\mathbf{r})\right]!. \tag{73}$$

The estimation of the DVF is then accomplished through the maximization of the following likelihood function

$$L(\mathbf{d}) = p(\mathbf{g}_1, \mathbf{g}_2; \mathbf{d}),$$

where $p(\cdot; \mathbf{d})$ represents the pdf parameterized by $\mathbf{d}$. This expression is difficult to evaluate because $\mathbf{g}_1$ and $\mathbf{g}_2$ are correlated. They become independent when conditioned on $\mathbf{f}$. Therefore, the method of conditioning is used such that $L(\mathbf{d})$ becomes

$$L(\mathbf{d}) = E_{\mathbf{f}} \{p(\mathbf{g}_1, \mathbf{g}_2|\mathbf{f}; \mathbf{d})\}$$

$$= \int_{\mathbf{f}} p(\mathbf{g}_1, \mathbf{g}_2|\mathbf{f}; \mathbf{d}) p(\mathbf{f}; \mathbf{d}) d\mathbf{f},$$

where $E_{\mathbf{f}}$ is the expectation operator with respect to $\mathbf{f}$. In this new form, however, the integral still cannot be evaluated[75] due to the doubly stochastic nature of the observations. Specifically, an exact expression involves the integration of the product of a Gaussian and a Poisson density, which has no closed form. The likelihood function can be evaluated when count-record data is available as shown in [73]. This is because a sample function density can be specified which describes the probability of obtaining a count-record data realization as a function of the position and time of detection. In turn, a likelihood function which is formed from this density function contains additional information with which to estimate parameters (such as the intensity function, Λ) that themselves are spatially and temporally varying through a maximization algorithm. But again, the imaging system has no means of acquiring information about the location of each photoevent. Consequently, a joint signal and DVF estimation approach is used where the maximization is performed using a block component search algorithm.

3.8.2. Iterative DVF and Signal Estimation

In light of the difficulties in the specification of a suitable likelihood function for maximization, the problem of displacement field estimation under quantum-limited conditions is formulated here by the joint estimation of the signal, $\mathbf{f}(\mathbf{r})$, and the displacement vector, $\mathbf{d}(\mathbf{r})$, at all locations $\mathbf{r} \in A$, from the two observed, degraded images, $\mathbf{g}_1$ and $\mathbf{g}_2$. This is a "mixed Fisher-Bayesian" likelihood method because of the presence of both deterministic and random quantities.[60] The reason for a joint estimation is fostered not only for the reasons cited in Section 3.8.1, but also by its ability to retain good quality estimates of the unknown displacement in terms of the mean square error despite the absence of knowledge of the signal.[71] This is accomplished through a maximization of the following likelihood function:

$$L(\mathbf{d}, \mathbf{f}|\mathbf{g}_1, \mathbf{g}_2).$$

Maximization of this likelihood function is equivalent to the maximization of the joint probability density function of the random vectors $\mathbf{f}$, $\mathbf{g}_1$, $\mathbf{g}_2$ given the deterministic field $\mathbf{d}$ upon removal of $p(\mathbf{d})$ and terms independent of $\mathbf{f}$ and $\mathbf{d}$ since

$$L(\mathbf{d}, \mathbf{f}|\mathbf{g}_1, \mathbf{g}_2) = p(\mathbf{d}, \mathbf{f}|\mathbf{g}_1, \mathbf{g}_2)$$

$$= \frac{p(\mathbf{d}, \mathbf{f}, \mathbf{g}_1, \mathbf{g}_2)}{p(\mathbf{g}_1, \mathbf{g}_2)}$$

$$= \frac{p(\mathbf{f}, \mathbf{g}_1, \mathbf{g}_2|\mathbf{d})p(\mathbf{d})}{p(\mathbf{g}_1, \mathbf{g}_2)}$$

$$\propto p(\mathbf{f}, \mathbf{g}_1, \mathbf{g}_2|\mathbf{d}).$$

Because of the monotonicity properties of the logarithmic function, the maximization of the likelihood function can be replaced by the maximization of the loglikelihood function:

$$\mathcal{L}(\mathbf{d}, \mathbf{f}|\mathbf{g}_1, \mathbf{g}_2) = \log p(\mathbf{f}, \mathbf{g}_1, \mathbf{g}_2|\mathbf{d})$$

$$= \log\left[p(\mathbf{g}_1, \mathbf{g}_2|\mathbf{f}, \mathbf{d})p(\mathbf{f}|\mathbf{d})\right].$$

Employing the property of independent increments processes,[66]

$$\mathcal{L}(\mathbf{d}, \mathbf{f}|\mathbf{g}_1, \mathbf{g}_2) = \log\left[p(\mathbf{g}_1|\mathbf{f}, \mathbf{d})p(\mathbf{g}_2|\mathbf{f}, \mathbf{d})p(\mathbf{f}|\mathbf{d})\right]$$

$$= \log\left[p(\mathbf{g}_1|\mathbf{f}, \mathbf{d})p(\mathbf{g}_2|\mathbf{f})p(\mathbf{f})\right]$$

$$= \log p(\mathbf{g}_1|\mathbf{f}, \mathbf{d}) + \log p(\mathbf{g}_2|\mathbf{f}) + \log p(\mathbf{f}), \quad (74)$$

where $\mathbf{g}_2$ is independent of $\mathbf{d}$ as given by Equation (73) and $\mathbf{f}$ is also independent of $\mathbf{d}$. The maximum *a posteriori* estimate of the unknown parameters is given by

$$\hat{\mathbf{f}}_{\text{MAP}}, \hat{\mathbf{d}}_{\text{MAP}} \leftarrow \arg\max_{\{\mathbf{f}, \mathbf{d}\}} \mathcal{L}(\mathbf{d}, \mathbf{f}|\mathbf{g}_1, \mathbf{g}_2).$$

Because $\mathbf{f}$ was assumed to be Gaussian and $\mathbf{d}$ is nonrandom, these estimates are equivalent to the maximum likelihood estimates and are referred to as ML estimates below.

In general, this multidimensional optimization problem is difficult to solve due to the complexity. Furthermore, it is not straightforward to take the Hessian of the likelihood function because of the nonlinear manner in which **d** appears. In order to alleviate this difficulty, a block component search algorithm is employed.[60] That is, a function of two variables is maximized by first keeping one of the variables constant and maximizing the function with respect to the other, followed by a subsequent maximization of the next variable in the same manner. A similar approach was utilized for variable time delay estimation for the Gaussian noise case in [63,77] This optimization strategy should achieve a local maximum of $\mathcal{L}(\mathbf{d}, \mathbf{f})$, but there is no guarantee that it will achieve a global maximum of $\mathcal{L}(\mathbf{d}, \mathbf{f})$.[60]

3.8.2.1. Estimation of the DVF

Specifically, if **f** were held fixed, the log-likelihood function in Equation (74) could then be written as

$$\mathcal{L}(\mathbf{d}, \mathbf{f}|\mathbf{g}_1, \mathbf{g}_2) = \mathcal{L}(\mathbf{d}|\mathbf{g}_1, \mathbf{g}_2)$$

$$= \log p(\mathbf{g}_1|\mathbf{f}, \mathbf{d}) + C,$$

where terms independent of **d** have been grouped together and represented by C. If a region, B, of the image is assumed to be translating uniformly with the common displacement vector, $\mathbf{d}(\mathbf{r}) = \mathbf{d}_B$, then the estimate of this displacement vector, using Equations (72) and (73), becomes

$$\hat{\mathbf{d}}_B \leftarrow \arg \max_{\mathbf{d}_B} \left[\log p(\mathbf{g}_1|\mathbf{f}, \mathbf{d}_B) \right]$$

$$= \arg \max_{\mathbf{d}_B} \left[\sum_{\mathbf{r} \in B} \lambda \mathbf{g}_1(\mathbf{r}) \ln \lambda \mathbf{f}(\mathbf{r} + \mathbf{d}_B) - \lambda \mathbf{f}(\mathbf{r} + \mathbf{d}_B) \right]$$

$$= \arg \max_{\mathbf{d}_B} \left[\lambda \sum_{\mathbf{r} \in B} \mathbf{g}_1(\mathbf{r}) \ln \lambda \mathbf{f}(\mathbf{r} + \mathbf{d}_B) - \mathbf{f}(\mathbf{r} + \mathbf{d}_B) \right]$$

$$= \arg \max_{\mathbf{d}_B} \left[\lambda \sum_{\mathbf{r} \in B} \mathbf{g}_1(\mathbf{r}) \left[\ln \lambda + \ln \mathbf{f}(\mathbf{r} + \mathbf{d}_B) \right] - \mathbf{f}(\mathbf{r} + \mathbf{d}_B) \right]$$

$$= \arg \max_{\mathbf{d}_B} \left[\sum_{\mathbf{r} \in B} \mathbf{g}_1(\mathbf{r}) \ln \mathbf{f}(\mathbf{r} + \mathbf{d}_B) - \mathbf{f}(\mathbf{r} + \mathbf{d}_B) \right]. \tag{75}$$

Note that if B is a square block and the maximization in Equation (75) is performed over all such individual blocks in the image, an algorithm similar to the block matching (BM) algorithm[65] results, but with a nonlinear maximization term. In other words, the maximization is done over a prespecified search area for the block B. However, it should be emphasized that, contrary to the BM algorithms in the literature, this estimator is derived based on a model for the underlying physical process.

3.8.2.2. Estimation of the intensity field

Similarly, if the displacement vector field, $\mathbf{d}$, is held fixed, a simpler solution for the estimate of the signal is possible. Specifically, the maximization problem reduces to one of estimating the signal given $\mathbf{g}_1, \mathbf{g}_2$ and $\mathbf{d}$, which compensates $\mathbf{g}_1$ to $\mathbf{g}_2$. In other words, there are two *motion-compensated* observations based on the knowledge of $\mathbf{d}$, as in the multiple input case of Section 3.4.1. Consequently, the maximum-likelihood estimate of the signal becomes

$$\hat{\mathbf{f}} \leftarrow \arg \max_{\mathbf{f}} p(\mathbf{g}_1, \mathbf{g}_2 | \mathbf{f}; \mathbf{d}) p(\mathbf{f}).$$

This is equivalent to the maximum *a posteriori* (MAP) estimate and also the minimum mean square error (MMSE) estimate of $\mathbf{f}$ because $\mathbf{f}$ was assumed to be Gaussian.[59] In general, this conditional mean is nonlinear. However, the same assumption used in Section 3.5 that the intensity estimator is locally linear at each pixel is made here. This is justified for the linear NMNV model which characterizes the image as a collection of Gaussians with distinctive local means and local variances at each pixel.

Using this assumption, the problem reduces to a total of M linear estimators, one at each pixel, for M pixels:

$$\hat{\mathbf{f}}(\mathbf{r}) = \gamma_1 \mathbf{g}_1(\mathbf{r} + \mathbf{d}(\mathbf{r})) + \gamma_2 \mathbf{g}_2(\mathbf{r}) + \gamma_0, \tag{76}$$

where the γ_i's are the optimal spatially varying coefficients giving the minimum mean square error. These optimal coefficients are given by Equation (14), renumbered here as a function of $\mathbf{d}$,

$$\gamma_0 = (1 - \gamma_1 - \gamma_2) E\{\mathbf{f}(\mathbf{r})\}$$

$$\gamma_1 = \frac{\sigma_{n_2}^2(\mathbf{r})\sigma_f^2(\mathbf{r})}{\sigma_f^2(\mathbf{r})\left[\sigma_{n_1}^2(\mathbf{r}+\mathbf{d}) + \sigma_{n_2}^2(\mathbf{r})\right] + \sigma_{n_1}^2(\mathbf{r}+\mathbf{d})\sigma_{n_2}^2(\mathbf{r})},$$

$$\gamma_2 = \frac{\sigma_{n_1}^2(\mathbf{r}+\mathbf{d})\sigma_f^2(\mathbf{r})}{\sigma_f^2(\mathbf{r})\left[\sigma_{n_1}^2(\mathbf{r}+\mathbf{d}) + \sigma_{n_2}^2(\mathbf{r})\right] + \sigma_{n_1}^2(\mathbf{r}+\mathbf{d})\sigma_{n_2}^2(\mathbf{r})}, \tag{77}$$

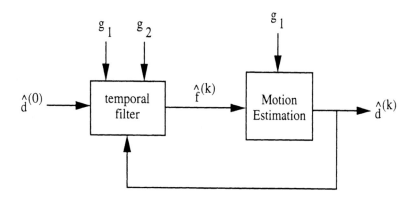

Figure 13. Iterative ML displacement field estimator.

where $\sigma_{n_1}^2(\mathbf{r})$ and $\sigma_{n_2}^2(\mathbf{r})$ are the variances of the nonstationary noise in frames 1 and 2, respectively, and $\sigma_f^2(\mathbf{r})$ is the local variance of the nonstationary signal, all at pixel location $\mathbf{r}$.

Consequently, the block component search algorithm iterates between Equation (75) and Equation (76) until an appropriate convergence criterion is met. In summary, the algorithm for displacement field estimation under quantum-limited conditions here is given by the following two stages:

$$\hat{\mathbf{d}}_B^{(k+1)} \leftarrow \arg\max_{\mathbf{d}_B} \left[\sum_{r \in B} \mathbf{g}_1(\mathbf{r}) \log \hat{\mathbf{f}}^{(k)}(\mathbf{r} + \mathbf{d_B}) - \hat{\mathbf{f}}^{(k)}(\mathbf{r} + \mathbf{d_B}) \right]$$

$$\hat{\mathbf{f}}^{(k+1)} = E\{\mathbf{f}|\mathbf{g_1}, \mathbf{g_2}; \hat{\mathbf{d}}_\mathbf{B}^{(k+1)}\}, \tag{78}$$

as shown in Figure 13.

3.8.3. Discussion

A novel approach to the estimation of the motion in signal-dependent noise problems has been described. A joint signal and displacement field estimator was derived under a maximum likelihood formulation to obtain a motion-compensation technique for image sequences corrupted by quantum mottle — a Poisson-distributed, signal-dependent noise source typical of that found in low-dose fluoroscopy images and low-light level video. The advantages of this formulation lies in the ability to develop model-based approaches derived from underlying physical processes. Preliminary experiments of simulated mottle on a phantom sequence and a sequence with real motion have demonstrated the increased robustness of this estimator in this type of noise, compared with conventional approaches.[16]

Current research focuses on developing iterative maximum *a posteriori* (MAP) estimators for the quantum-limited imaging conditions by incorporating prior knowledge of the displacement field.[8,12] Hierarchical block-based estimators are also being considered since it is well known that improved resolution of the DVF can be expected by such modeling. In addition, the use of nonlinear signal estimators such as those described in Section 3.7 can be expected to improve the iterates generated.[15]

3.9. CONCLUSIONS

This chapter was concerned with the problem of image sequence filtering with quantum-limited scenes. This work was motivated in part by the need for temporal filtering methods in low dose fluoroscopy to improve image quality degraded as a result of intentionally lowering X-ray dosages traditionally used in practice.

A generalization of the stochastic noise model often used in quantum-limited images was proposed in this chapter and shown to be extendable to image sequences. From this noise model, a set of motion-compensated temporal filters was derived and compared to existing spatial filtering methods which use no correlation between frames. Specifically, a batch-type temporal filter and its recursive implementation were considered here.

Some preliminary work in new approaches to filtering and displacement field estimation in quantum mottle were described. Specifically, a nonlinear filter based on a Volterra expansion and a motion estimator derived using physical principles were proposed. These methods have looked promising for nonclinical and may seem to be well suited for angiography applications as well.

3.10. APPENDIX: DERIVATION OF HIGHER ORDER NOISE STATISTICS

Recall the observation equation

$$g(\mathbf{r}) = f(\mathbf{r}) + n_g(\mathbf{r}). \tag{79}$$

For a zero-mean Poisson distributed noise,

$$E\{n_g(\mathbf{r})\} = 0 \tag{80}$$

and

$$\sigma_{n_g}^2(\mathbf{r}) = E\{n_g^2(\mathbf{r})\} = \frac{1}{\lambda}E\{f\}. \tag{81}$$

To find the third order moment of the noise, let

$$n_g^3(\mathbf{r}) = [g(\mathbf{r}) - f(\mathbf{r})]^3 . \tag{82}$$

Then

$$E\{n_g^3(\mathbf{r})\} = E\{g^3(\mathbf{r})\} - 3E\{g^2(\mathbf{r})f(\mathbf{r})\} + 3E\{g(\mathbf{r})f^2(\mathbf{r})\} - E\{f^3(\mathbf{r})\}. \tag{83}$$

The analysis can be separated into three parts. First

$$E\{g^2 f\} = E\{f E\{g^2 | f\}\}$$

$$= \frac{1}{\lambda^2}E\{f E\{N^2 | f\}\}$$

$$= \frac{1}{\lambda^2}E\left\{f\left[\lambda f + \lambda^2 f^2\right]\right\}$$

$$= \frac{1}{\lambda}E\{f^2\} + E\{f^3\}. \tag{84}$$

Next,

$$E\{g^3\} = \frac{1}{\lambda^3}E\{N^3\}$$

$$= \frac{1}{\lambda^3}E\{E\{N^3 | f\}\}$$

$$= \frac{1}{\lambda^3}E\left\{\int N^2 p(N | f)dN\right\}$$

$$= \frac{1}{\lambda^3}E\{\lambda f + 3(\lambda f)^2 + (\lambda f)^3\}$$

$$= \frac{1}{\lambda^2}E\{f\} + \frac{3}{\lambda}E\{f^2\} + E\{f^3\}. \tag{85}$$

The computation of the fourth step is given by the recursion relation for Poisson moments with parameter a,[46,66] that is,

$$m_{n+1}(a) = a\left[m_n(a) + m'_n(a)\right] \tag{86}$$

where $m_n(a)$ is the n-th order conditional moment of N here. Furthermore, it can be shown that the conditional moment of g is given by a modified recursion relation

$$E\{g^{n+1}|f\} = f\left[E\{g^n|f\} + \frac{1}{\lambda}\nabla_g E\{g^n|f\}\right]. \tag{87}$$

Finally,

$$E\{gf^2\} = E\{f^2 E\{N|f\}\}$$

$$= \frac{1}{\lambda}E\{f^2 E\{N|f\}\}$$

$$= \frac{1}{\lambda}E\{f^2(\lambda f)\}$$

$$= E\{f^3\}. \tag{88}$$

Therefore,

$$E\{n_g^3\} = \frac{1}{\lambda^2}E\{f\} + \frac{3}{\lambda}E\{f^2\} + E\{f^3\}$$

$$- 3\left[\frac{1}{\lambda}E\{f^2\} + E\{f^3\}\right] + 3E\{f^3\} - E\{f^3\}$$

$$= \frac{1}{\lambda^2}E\{f\}. \tag{89}$$

To find the fourth order moment of the noise, let

$$n^4(\mathbf{r}) = [g(\mathbf{r}) - f(\mathbf{r})]^4. \tag{90}$$

Then

$$E\{n_g^4(\mathbf{r})\} = E\{g^4(\mathbf{r})\} - 4E\{g^3(\mathbf{r})f(\mathbf{r})\} + 6E\{g^2(\mathbf{r})f^2(\mathbf{r})\}$$

$$- 4E\{g(\mathbf{r})f^3(\mathbf{r})\} + E\{f^4(\mathbf{r})\}. \tag{91}$$

Again, the analysis is broken into 4 parts. First,

$$E\{g^4\} = \frac{1}{\lambda^4} E\{N^4\}$$

$$= \frac{1}{\lambda^4} E\{E\{N^4|f\}\}$$

$$= \frac{1}{\lambda^4} E\left\{\int N^4 p(N|f) dN\right\}$$

$$= \frac{1}{\lambda^4} E\{(\lambda f)^4 + 6(\lambda f)^3 + 7(\lambda f)^2 + (\lambda f)\}$$

$$= E\{f^4\} + \frac{6}{\lambda} E\{f^3\} + \frac{7}{\lambda^2} E\{f^2\} + \frac{1}{\lambda^3} E\{f\} \qquad (92)$$

where the computation of the fourth step is again given by the recursion relation in Equation (86), and

$$E\{g^3 f\} = E\{f E\{g^3|f\}\}$$

$$= \frac{1}{\lambda^3} E\{f E\{N^3|f\}\}$$

$$= \frac{1}{\lambda^3} E\left\{f \left[(\lambda f) + 3(\lambda f)^2 + (\lambda f)^3\right]\right\}$$

$$= \frac{1}{\lambda^2} E\{f^2\} + \frac{3}{\lambda} E\{f^3\} + E\{f^4\}. \qquad (93)$$

Then,

$$E\{g^2 f^2\} = E\{f^2 E\{g^2|f\}\}$$

$$= \frac{1}{\lambda^2} E\{f^2 E\{N^2|f\}\}$$

$$= \frac{1}{\lambda^2} E\left\{f^2 \left[\lambda f + \lambda^2 f^2\right]\right\}$$

$$= \frac{1}{\lambda} E\{f^3\} + E\{f^4\}. \qquad (94)$$

Finally,

$$E\{gf^3\} = E\{f^3 E\{g|f\}\}$$

$$= \frac{1}{\lambda} E\{f^3 E\{N|f\}\}$$

$$= \frac{1}{\lambda} E\{f^3 (\lambda f)\}$$

$$= E\{f^4\}. \tag{95}$$

Summing the terms together,

$$E\{n_g^4\} = E\{f^4\} + \frac{6}{\lambda} E\{f^3\} + \frac{7}{\lambda^2} E\{f^2\} + \frac{1}{\lambda^3} E\{f\}$$

$$- 4E\{f^4\} - \frac{12}{\lambda} E\{f^3\} - \frac{4}{\lambda^2} E\{f^2\}$$

$$+ 6E\{f^4\} + \frac{6}{\lambda} E\{f^3\} - 4E\{f^4\} + E\{f^4\}$$

$$= \frac{1}{\lambda^3} E\{f\} + \frac{3}{\lambda^2} E\{f^2\}. \tag{96}$$

3.11. REFERENCES

1. Abdelqader, I.M. and S.A. Rajala, 1993, *Proc. ICASSP*, **V**, 209–212.
2. Anderson, J. M. and G.B. Giannakis, 1991, *Proc. ICASSP*, **4**, 2721–2724.
3. Antoniadis, N. and A. O. Hero, 1992, *Proc. ICASSP*, **5**, 289–292.
4. Biemond, J., L. Looijenga, D.E. Boekee and R.H.J.M. Plompen, 1987, *Signal Processing*, **13**, 399–412.
5. Brailean, J.C. and A.K. Katsaggelos, 1992, *Proc. EUSIPCO*, **3**, 1319–1322.
6. Brailean, J.C. and A.K. Katsaggelos, 1993, *Proc. ICASSP*, **V**, 273–276.
7. Brailean, J.C. and A.K. Katsaggelos, 1995, *IEEE Trans. Image Processing*, **4**, 416–429.
8. Brailean, J.C., C.L. Chan and A.K. Katsaggelos, 1995, *Proc SPIE, to appear*.
9. Brody, W.R., 1984, *Digital Radiography*, (Raven Press, New York).
10. Chan, C.L., A.K. Katsaggelos and A.V. Sahakian, 1992, *Proc. SPIE*, **1818**, 290–298.
11. Chan, C.L., A.K. Katsaggelos and A.V. Sahakian, 1993, *IEEE Trans. Med. Imaging*, **12**, 610–621.
12. Chan, C.L., A.K. Katsaggelos and A.V. Sahakian, 1993, *Journ. of Visual Comm. and Image Repr.*, **4**, 349–363.
13. Chan, C.L., B.J. Sullivan, A.V. Sahakian, A.K. Katsaggelos, S. Swiryn, D.C. Hueter and T. Frohlich, 1990, *Proc. SPIE*, **1245**, 104–110.
14. Chan, C.L., B.J. Sullivan, A.V. Sahakian, A.K. Katsaggelos, T. Frohlich and E. Byrom, 1991, *Proc. SPIE*, **1450**, 208–217.
15. Chan, C.L., J.C. Brailean, A.K. Katsaggelos and A.V. Sahakian, 1993, *Proc. SPIE*, **2094**, 396–407.

16. Chan, C.L. and A.K. Katsaggelos, 1995, *IEEE Trans. Image Processing*, **4**, 743–751.
17. Chan, C.L., A.K. Katsaggelos and A.V. Sahakian, 1995, *IEEE Trans. Image Processing*, **4**, 1328–1333.
18. Chen, Y., 1989, *IEEE Trans. Aero. and Elect. Sys.*, **25**, 343–350.
19. Dempster, A.P., N. Laird and D. Rubin, 1977, *J. Royal Statistical Society B*, **39**, 1–37.
20. Dubois, E. and S. Sabri, 1984, *IEEE Trans. Comm.*, **32**, 821–826.
21. Efstratiadis, S.N. and A.K. Katsaggelos, 1993, *IEEE Trans. Image Processing*, **2**, 341–352.
22. Efstratiadis, S.N. and A.K. Katsaggelos, 1992, *IEEE Trans. Circuits, Syst., and Video Techn.*, **2**, 334–346.
23. Enzmann, D.R., W.T. Djang, S.J. Riederer, W.F. Collins, A. Hall, G.S. Keyes and W.R. Brody, 1983, *Radiology*, **146**, 669-676.
24. Eykhoff, P., 1963, *IEEE Trans. Auto. Control*, **8**, 347–357.
25. Fam, B.W. and S.L. Olsen, 1987, *Proc. SPIE*, **767**, 416–424.
26. Fishman, P.M. and D.L. Snyder, 1976, *IEEE Trans. Info. Theory*, **22**, 257–274.
27. Frieden, B.R., 1987, *Applied Optics*, **26**, 1755–1764.
28. Friedlander, B. and B. Porat, 1990, *IEEE Trans. Auto. Control*, **35**, 27–35.
29. Fritz, S.L., S.E. Mirvis, S.O. Pais and S. Roys, 1988, *Med. Phys.*, **15**, 600–603.
30. Galatsanos, N.P. and R.T. Chin, 1989, *IEEE Trans. Acoust., Speech, Signal Proc.*, **37**, 415–421.
31. Galatsanos, N.P., A.K. Katsaggelos, R.T. Chin and A.D. Hillery, 1991, *IEEE Trans. Signal Proc.*, **39**, 2222–2236.
32. Garth, L.M. and Y. Bresler, 1993, *Proc. ICASSP*, **IV**, 208–211.
33. Geman, S. and D. Geman, 1984, *IEEE Trans. Patt. Anal. and Mach. Intel.*, **6**, 721–741.
34. Ghiglia, D., 1982, *Journ. Opt. Soc. Amer. A*, **1**, 398–402.
35. Goldberg, H.L., *et al.*, 1986, *Chest*, **90**, 793–797.
36. Haykin, S., 1991, *Adaptive Filter Theory*, (Prentice-Hall, Englewood Cliffs), 2nd ed.
37. Hayworth, M., B.R. Frieden and H. Roehrig, 1987, *Proc. SPIE*, **767**, 471–478.
38. Hero, A.O., 1989, *IEEE Trans. Info. Theory*, **35**, 843–858.
39. Hero, A.O., 1991, *IEEE Trans. Info. Theory*, **37**, 92–106.
40. Holmes, T.J., 1992, *Journ. Opt. Soc. Amer. A*, **9**, 1052–1061.
41. Huang, T.S. and R.V. Tsai, 1981, in *Image Sequence Analysis*, (Springer-Verlag, Berlin), 104–124.
42. Hull, D.M., C.S. Peskin, A.M. Rabinowitz, J.P. Wexler and M.D. Blaufox, 1990, *Phys. Med. Biol.*, **35**, 1641–1662.
43. Hunt, B.R. and O. Kubler, 1984, *IEEE Trans. Acoust., Speech, Signal Proc.*, **32**, 592–600.
44. Jeng, F.-C. and J.W. Woods, 1988, *IEEE Trans. Acoust., Speech, Signal Proc.*, **36**, 1305–1312.
45. Jiang, S.S. and A.A. Sawchuk, 1986, *Appl. Opt.*, **25**, 2326–2337.
46. Johnson, N.L. and S. Kotz, 1969, *Discrete Distributions*, New York: Wiley-Interscience.
47. Kalivas, D.S. and A.A. Sawchuk, 1990, *Proc. ICASSP*, **4**, 2121–2125.
48. Kasturi, R., J.F. Walkup and T.F. Krile, 1985, *IEEE Trans. Syst., Man, Cyber.*, **15**, 352–359.
49. Katsaggelos, A.K., 1990, *Journ. Visual Comm. and Image Rep.*, **1**, 93–103.
50. Katsaggelos, A.K., J.N. Driessen, S.N. Efstratiadis and R. Lagendijk, 1989, *Proc. SPIE*, **1199**, 61–70.
51. Katsaggelos, A.K., R.P. Kleihorst, S.N. Efstratiadis and R.L. Lagendijk, 1991, *Proc. SPIE*, **1606**, 716–727.
52. Koh, T. and E.J. Powers, 1995, *IEEE Trans. Acoust., Speech, Signal Proc.*, **33**, 1445–1455.
53. Konrad, J. and E. Dubois, 1992, *IEEE Trans. Patt. Anal. and Mach. Intel.*, **14**, 910–927.
54. Kuan, D.T., A.A. Sawchuk, T.C. Strand and P. Chavel, 1985, *IEEE Trans. Patt. Anal. Mach. Intel.*, **7**, 653–665.
55. Lefree, M.T., S.B. Simon, M.L. Sanz, R.A. Vogel and G.B.J. Mancini, 1988, in *Clinical Applications of Cardiac Digital Angiography*, (Raven Press, New York), 219–237.
56. Lo, C.M. and A.A. Sawchuk, 1979, *Proc. SPIE*, **207**, 84–95.
57. Macovski, A., 1983, *Medical Imaging Systems*, (Prentice-Hall, Englewood Cliffs).

58. Martinez, D.M., 1986, *Ph.D. dissertation, Massachusetts Institute of Technology*.
59. Maybeck, P.S. 1979, *Stochastic models, estimation, and control*, vol. 1, San Diego: Academic Press, Inc.
60. Mendel, J.M., 1990, *Maximum-Likelihood Deconvolution: A Journey into Model-Based Signal Processing*, New York: Springer-Verlag.
61. Mort, M.S. and M.D. Srinath, 1988, *Proc. SPIE*, **974**, 38–44.
62. Morris, G.M. 1984, *Journ. Opt. Soc. Amer. A*, **1**, 482–488.
63. Namazi, N.M. and J.A. Stuller, 1987, *IEEE Trans. Acoust., Speech, Signal Proc.*, **35**, 1649–1660.
64. Namazi, N.M. and C.H. Lee, 1990, *IEEE Trans. Acoust., Speech, Signal Proc.*, **38**, 364–366.
65. Netravali, A.N. and B.G. Haskell, 1988, *Digital Pictures – Representation and Compression*, (Plenum Press, New York).
66. Papoulis, A., 1984, *Probability, Random Variables, and Stochastic Processes*, (McGraw-Hill, New York), 2nd Ed.
67. Parker, D.L., P.D. Clayton, L.R. Tarbox and P.L. VonBehren, 1983, *Proc. SPIE*, **419**, 102–110.
68. Picinbono, B. and P. Duvaut, 1988, *IEEE Trans. Info. Theory*, **34**, 304–311.
69. Picinbono, B., 1989, *Proc Workshop on Higher Order Spectral Analysis, Vail, Colorado*, 62–67.
70. Pohlig, S.C., 1989, *IEEE Trans. Aero. and Elect. Sys.*, **25**, 56–63.
71. Segal, M., E. Weinstein and B.R. Musicus, 1991, *IEEE Trans. Signal Proc.*, **39**, 1–16.
72. Singh, A., 1992, *Proc. SPIE*, **1660**, 288–298.
73. Slocumb, B.J. and D.L. Snyder, 1990, *Proc. SPIE*, **1304**, 165–176.
74. Snyder, D.L. and T.J. Schulz, 1990, *Journ. Opt. Soc. Amer. A*, **7**, 1251–1265.
75. Snyder, D.L. and M.I. Miller, 1991, *Random Point Processes in Time and Space*, (Springer-Verlag, New York), 2nd ed.
76. Sprawls, P., 1987, *Physical Principles of Medical Imaging*, (Aspen Publishers, Inc., Maryland).
77. Stuller, J.A., 1987, *IEEE Trans. on Acoust., Speech, Signal Proc.*, **35**, 300–313.
78. Venot, A. and V. LeClerc, 1984, *IEEE Trans. Med. Imaging*, **3**, 179–186.
79. Zuiderveld, K.J., B.M. ter Haar Romeny and M.A. Viergever, 1989, *Proc. SPIE*, **1137**, 22–30.

4 AUTOMATED ANALYSIS OF CORONARY ANGIOGRAMS*

MILAN SONKA[†] and STEVE M. COLLINS

*Departments of Electrical and Computer Engineering, and Radiology
The University of Iowa, Iowa City, IA 52242, USA*

4.1. INTRODUCTION

Each year about 1.5 million people in the United States with coronary artery disease suffer myocardial infarction.[1] The death rate from coronary artery disease is in excess of 500,000 per year. In the 35 years since 1959 when Sones introduced selective catheterization of the coronary arteries, coronary angiography has achieved a preeminent position in the armamentarium of the physician caring for the cardiac patient.[2] Assessment of coronary arterial geometry is central to the diagnosis of coronary artery disease, to decisions about pharmacological therapy or coronary artery revascularization with transluminal coronary angioplasty or coronary artery bypass surgery,[3] to judgments about the short and long-term outcome of revascularization procedures, and to assessment of patient prognosis. Although a variety of cardiac imaging techniques are under active development, selective coronary arteriography is the only method capable of accurately depicting the details of coronary anatomy[2] (Figure 1). Accordingly, coronary angiography has

---

*Portions reprinted, with permission, from IEEE Transactions on Medical Imaging, Volume 12, pages 588–599, September 1993; IEEE Transactions on Medical Imaging, Volume 14, pages 151–161, March 1995. ©1993, 1995 IEEE.

[†]Correspondence: Milan Sonka, Department of Electrical and Computer Engineering, University of Iowa, Iowa City, Iowa, 52242. Phone: (319)-335-6052; Fax: (319)-335-6028; e-mail: milan-sonka@uiowa.edu.

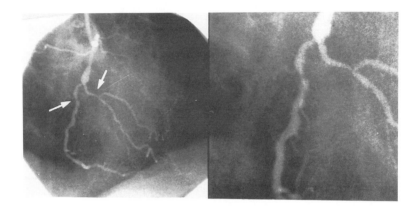

Figure 1. Coronary angiograms. (left) Angiogram of the coronary tree. Stenotic vessel is depicted by arrow. (right) Stenotic vessel segment, magnified.

maintained a pivotal role in the evaluation and treatment of patients with coronary disease[4] and hundreds of thousands of coronary angiograms are performed every year in the United States.

The vast majority of these angiograms are interpreted visually. Visual assessment of the severity of coronary disease is associated with very substantial inter- and intra-observer variability.[5-7] Moreover, visual interpretation of coronary angiograms does not allow accurate assessment of the physiological significance of coronary obstructions.[8] The shortcomings of visual analysis have prompted leading clinical investigators to call for the use of quantitative coronary angiography for assessing coronary obstruction severity in routine patient care.[3,9-12] A very substantial amount of research has been directed at the development of semi-automated and automated methods for defining coronary arterial borders and calculating indices of lesion severity and physiologic significance.[13-25] As a result, automated approaches were developed to identify vessel borders and calculate indices of stenosis severity from coronary angiograms. Automated coronary border detection has become a standard component of experimental studies evaluating diagnostic approaches to detecting coronary disease,[26] assessing the efficacy of surgical, mechanical and pharmacological interventional therapeutic procedures,[4,27] and studying the progression and regression of coronary atherosclerosis.[28-30] To date, automated border detection methods have seen limited application in routine clinical care and most patient management decisions are based on visual estimates of percent diameter stenosis.[11] Factors that have contributed to the limited acceptance of automated methods include the need for specialized equipment and software, the time-consuming nature of some methods, and problems in reliably detecting vessel borders.

Despite the widely recognized limitations of visual assessment of lesion severity, most patient management decisions continue to be based on visual assessment of percent diameter stenosis.[3,11] An important reason for the poor clinical acceptance of quantitative coronary angiography is its limited reliability in clinical use. Current automated methods for identifying vessel borders from coronary angiograms often fail to accurately identify vessel borders, particularly when applied to the routine analysis of clinical angiograms. The presence of poor contrast, branching vessels, and overlapping or adjacent structures near the vessel segment of interest all present difficulties for automated methods.

4.2. APPROACHES TO ANALYSIS OF CORONARY ANGIOGRAMS

Assessment of coronary obstruction severity by visual estimation of percent diameter stenosis from angiograms suffers from poor inter- and intra-observer reproducibility.[5-7] The limited reproducibility of visual assessment is a particular concern in the evaluation of risk factor modifications and pharmacologic and mechanical interventions where accurate estimates of stenosis regression or progression are required. Visual estimates also demonstrate systematic errors with visual estimates of percent diameter stenosis being larger than quantitative estimates by as much as 30 percentage points.[31] Visual interpretation significantly overestimates lesion severity before angioplasty and underestimates stenosis severity after angioplasty.[32] These systematic errors cannot be attributed to the experience of the observer.[32] The widely recognized shortcomings of visual evaluation of coronary angiograms have led to substantial research directed at development of automated methods to assess coronary artery geometry.[33]

4.2.1. Videodensitometric Approaches

Automated methods for evaluation of coronary lesion severity can be divided into geometric[13-25] and videodensitometric approaches. Videodensitometric approaches are based on the density of contrast material in the vessel lumen and allow estimation of lumen cross-sectional area from a single angiographic view.[19,34-38] Importantly, these approaches do not depend on assumptions about the cross-sectional shape of the vessel and do not require precise definition of the vessel borders.[39] Thus, videodensitometric approaches should in theory be of particular value following percutaneous transluminal angioplasty when indistinct borders and irregularly shaped and eccentric stenoses are common.[40−42] In practice, videodensitometric approaches are limited by numerous sources of error. These include beam hardening, scatter, veiling glare, vessel foreshortening, contributions from background, and incomplete mixing of contrast.[28,43,44] As a result, reproducibility of videodensitometric methods may be less than that for geometric methods[45] and estimates of lumen area obtained in multiple views may not agree.[46] Perhaps accordingly, more research has been directed at the development of automated border detection methods than on videodensitometric methods. It is of course possible and even advantageous to combine border detection and videodensitometric approaches.[16,19,41,47]

4.2.2. Geometric Approaches

Conventional geometric approaches to evaluation of coronary geometry are based on automated detection of individual coronary borders and on using data from two or more angiographic projections to reconstruct a three-dimensional representation of coronary lesion size and shape. An example of this latter approach is the Brown-Dodge method of quantitative coronary arteriography.[13] This method has been widely used and extensively validated[13,48−50] and it was employed as an independent standard in many later studies. A great variety of methods for automated detection of coronary borders have been introduced.[13−25,51] In general, these methods detect coronary borders by identifying image pixels with large gradients. Such edge detection is typically a local process in that the position of the detected edge depends largely on local image characteristics. Although this approach works well in high-quality images, it ignores global information that is very useful in detecting local border position in images of intermediate or poor quality. Reiber *et al.* were the first to report a coronary border detection technique that identified a border that in a global sense was optimal.[15] Computer identification of optimal coronary borders is typically based on 2-D graph searching principles.[20] An optimal border can be defined as the border that in an overall sense had the greatest likelihood of corresponding to the actual coronary border. Parker and associates have developed a method based on dynamic programming that also identifies an optimal border.[52] Related approaches that are not restricted to defining the coronary border as a sequence of points, one per profile, have been reported.[22,53,54]

Although the anatomical characteristics of a coronary obstruction are of interest to the clinician, it is the physiological consequences of the obstruction that are important in arriving at decisions with respect to patient management. Minimal lumen diameters derived from automatically-identified coronary borders have been used to assess obstruction severity.[18−20,55] This approach is motivated by the fact that the minimal dimension of a stenosis is the single most important factor in determining the hemodynamic consequence of an obstruction.[28] Nonetheless, such methods fail to take into account important stenosis characteristics (normal area, stenotic area, length of lesion, entrance and exit angles) that can have functional consequences. An excellent example of an automated method that incorporates all of the vessel dimensions and predicts coronary flow reserve is that reported by Kirkeeide et al.[16] This method combines automated border detection and videodensitometry together with fluid dynamic principles to provide a single integrated functional measure of lesion severity.[56]

4.3. RELIABILITY OF QUANTITATIVE CORONARY ANGIOGRAPHY

The substantial research on quantitative coronary angiography has been motivated by two factors. The first is the extremely important role that assessment of coronary arterial geometry plays in the diagnosis and treatment of cardiovascular disease. With the dramatic expansion of interventional procedures for treating coronary disease in the catheterization laboratory, the need for reliable and readily available measures of lumen geometry has become ever more pressing.[4] Unfortunately, the standard deviation in visual estimation of percent stenosis is about 18% and a major disagreement occurs between readers in about 31% of vessels.[7] Illustrative of the poor reproducibility of visual analysis is the finding in the Coronary Artery Surgery Study that when one angiographer reported a stenosis of 50% diameter narrowing or more in the left main coronary artery, a second angiographer reported no lesion in 19% of cases.[57] Moreover, visual assessments are often inaccurate as demonstrated by comparisons with post-mortem anatomy.[58] Lesions with greater than 50% narrowing are overestimated by 15% to 30% diameter stenosis units.[3,4,32] Lesions below 50% narrowing tend to be underestimated. This leads to very substantial overestimation of the improvement in lumen diameter resulting from angioplasty.[32] Gould calls attention to the 189% error in assessing the average benefit of coronary angioplasty that results from inaccurate visual assessment of pre- and post-angioplasty percent stenosis.[10] Finally, visual estimates of percent diameter stenosis correlate poorly with direct measures of the physiologic significance of coronary obstructions.[8]

As a result of the shortcomings of visual analysis of coronary angiograms, use of quantitative coronary angiography in scientific studies and clinical trials has become the accepted standard. However, quantitative coronary angiography has not achieved widespread acceptance or use in routine patient care.[3,11] There are several explanations for the lack of acceptance of quantitative coronary angiography methods. Some methods are time consuming and require specialized equipment and/or expertise. This is a serious obstacle to routine clinical use since ease and speed of use are essential in a clinical setting.[4] No consensus has developed as to the best analysis algorithms.[4,33] Only a few border detection methods have been carefully validated *in vivo* by comparison to independent geometric and physiologic standards.[16,19,20,59] While automated border detection methods yield excellent results in investigational settings when applied to high quality images of vessel segments free of vessel overlap and other confounding variables, they often fail when applied to unselected vessel segments in a clinical setting. The limited reliability of quantitative coronary angiography methods in the clinical setting has severely impeded the routine use of these techniques.

Gurley *et al.* recently examined the suitability of quantitative coronary angiography for routine clinical use.[60] They analyzed 38 stenoses in digital angiograms from 25 consecutive patients using a commercially available analysis system.[61] Only definite lesions, defined as vessel segments visually determined by four independent observers to have lumen diameter reductions exceeding 50%, were analyzed. Quantitative coronary angiography successfully traced 20 stenoses but failed in 18/38 stenoses or 48%. The failures were attributed to stenosis at a bifurcation (72%), diffuse disease with no normal reference segment (44%), excessive vessel tortuosity or overlap (22%), and poor image contrast or under penetration (28%). Gurley *et al.* concluded that quantitative coronary angiography is unsuitable for routine clinical use and that a practical method of objectively assessing stenosis severity in the clinical setting remains to be developed.[61] Although details as to what constituted an analysis failure were not given and their results may not generalize to other quantitative coronary angiography techniques, clearly the reservations about quantitative coronary angiography expressed by these authors are shared by many clinicians. The critical need for robust quantitative coronary angiography methods and the substantial failure rate of current border detection methods form the impetus for development of robust knowledge-based approaches to coronary border detection.

4.4. BORDER DETECTION AS GRAPH SEARCHING

Graph searching is a standard technique of image segmentation and is particularly useful if borders of thin elongated objects like vessels are to be detected.[62] For graph construction, the edge image is resampled perpendicular to the vessel centerline to "straighten" the artery. The centerline becomes a straight line and the graph consists of a rectangular grid of nodes corresponding to pixels in the straightened image. A profile is defined as a set of nodes perpendicular to the straightened centerline. A cost is associated with each node that is inversely related to the edge strength of the corresponding pixel. A path through the graph connecting pixels at one end of the vessel (start nodes) to pixels at the other end (end nodes) corresponds to a possible coronary border. The graph searching technique determines the minimum cost path or optimal border. The cost function $f(\mathbf{x}_i)$ for a path containing a particular node $\mathbf{x}_i$ on the profile i typically consists of two components; an estimate $\tilde{g}(\mathbf{x}_i)$ of the minimum cost partial path between a starting node $\mathbf{x}_1$ and $\mathbf{x}_i$, and an estimate $\tilde{h}(\mathbf{x}_i)$ of the minimum cost partial path between $\mathbf{x}_i$ and an end node $\mathbf{x}_E$. The cost $\tilde{g}(\mathbf{x}_i)$ is the sum of costs associated with the nodes that are on the path. If the estimate $\tilde{h}(\mathbf{x}_i)$ is not considered (i.e., $\tilde{h}(\mathbf{x}_i) = 0$), no heuristic is included in the algorithm and a uniform-cost search is done (standard graph searching method). Although a uniform cost search guarantees that the optimal border (i.e., minimum cost path) will be found, a large number of paths must be examined.

One way to increase the search efficiency is to avoid examining paths that are far (in terms of cost) from the path that is ultimately determined to be optimal. If the cost of the minimum cost node on each profile is subtracted from the cost of each node on the profile, search efficiency is improved. We refer to this approach as the lower bound method. In effect, this shifts the range of costs associated with nodes on a given profile from

$$\min_k \{c(k, i)\} \le c(k, i) \le \max_k \{c(k, i)\}$$

to

$$0 \le c_{LB}(k, i) \le [\max_k \{c(k, i)\} - \min_k \{c(k, i)\}]$$

where $c(k, i)$ is the cost of the k-th node on the i-th profile and $c_{LB}(k, i)$ is the new lower bound cost of the node. It can be shown that the borders detected using the lower bound and conventional methods are exactly the same.

Additional increases in search efficiency can be achieved if $\tilde{h}(\mathbf{x}_i) > 0$. The minimum cost path identification can be guaranteed only if $\tilde{h}(\mathbf{x}_i) \le h(\mathbf{x}_i)$, where $h(\mathbf{x}_i)$ is the actual cost of the minimum cost partial path from $\mathbf{x}_i$ to $\mathbf{x}_N$. The closer the estimate $\tilde{h}(\mathbf{x}_i)$ is to $h(\mathbf{x}_i)$, the greater the efficiency of the search. The problem is that $h(\mathbf{x}_i)$ is not known beforehand. Should $\tilde{h}(\mathbf{x}_i)$ exceed $h(\mathbf{x}_i)$, detection of the optimal border is not guaranteed but search efficiency will be high since the search can be stopped before the optimum is found. Further details on heuristic graph searching image segmentation techniques are available in [62].

Dynamic programming represents another approach to optimal graph searching and is based on the principle of optimality.[63−65] It searches for optima of functions in which not all variables are simultaneously interrelated. The main idea of the principle of optimality is: whatever the path to the node N was, there exists an optimal path between N and the *end_point*. In other words, if the optimal path *start_point – end_point* goes through N then both its parts *start_point – N* and *N – end_point* are also optimal.

It has been shown that heuristic search may be more efficient than dynamic programming for finding a path between two nodes in a graph.[66] Further, heuristic graph search does not require explicit definition of the graph. However, dynamic programming presents an efficient way of simultaneous search for optimal paths from multiple starting and ending points. If these points are not known, dynamic programming is probably a better choice. Nevertheless, which approach is more efficient for a particular problem depends on evaluation functions and on the quality of heuristics for heuristic graph search. A comparison between dynamic programming and heuristic search efficiency can be found in [67].

4.5. CONVENTIONAL CORONARY BORDER DETECTION

Tremendous investigative effort has been devoted to the development of automated methods for evaluating coronary artery anatomy. Coronary border detection approaches traditionally consist of a number of steps:

1. observer identification of the vessel segment of interest;
2. application of an edge operator to derive an edge image;
3. geometric warping of the edge image;
4. construction of a directed graph and optimal border identification; and
5. mapping of the detected borders back into the original image space and calculation of a diameter function.

Many conventional geometric methods presented in Section 4.2.2 follow the above processing strategy. The method introduced in [20] can be considered a typical representative of such conventional methods. Below, we describe the approach to border detection reported by Fleagle *et al.*

4.5.1. Image Preprocessing

Following digitization of an optically magnified cine frame into an 8-bit 512×512 image matrix (resolution in object plane of about 60 μm/pixel), the centerline of the vessel segment of interest is interactively defined by an observer. The observer also enters two points, one on either side of the

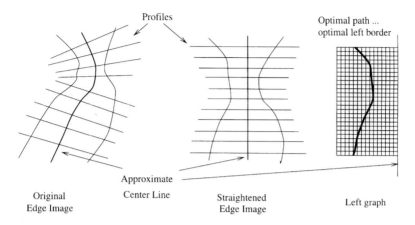

Figure 2. Illustration of the geometric warping applied to the edge image. The edge image is resampled along profile lines perpendicular to the vessel centerline in the original image space so as to produce a straightened artery in the resampled space. A two-dimensional graph is constructed from each half-plane of the straightened edge image.

vessel, which together with the vessel centerline define the image region of interest within which the vessel segment is located. The defined centerline only approximates the actual vessel centerline and is heavily smoothed.

A two-dimensional edge operator is then applied to the digitized image to produce an edge image (Figure 3a). The utilized edge operator is a weighted combination of a Sobel operator and a Marr-Hildreth operator. The Sobel operator uses an 11×11 mask and approximates the first derivative of image intensity. The Marr-Hildreth operator uses a 21×21 mask and approximates the second derivative of image intensity. It is reasonably well accepted that a combination of first and second derivative edge operators produces an accurate estimate of coronary edge position.[24,28,43] In [20], the mask sizes and relative weights were determined empirically from phantom studies.

For computational convenience, the edge image is resampled (on a square grid with one-pixel spacing and using interpolation) along profiles perpendicular to the centerline to "straighten" the artery (Figure 2). The straightened edge image is smoothed in the direction parallel to the vessel centerline.

4.5.2. Identification of Individual Borders

As described in Section 4.4, heuristic graph search is used to identify optimal coronary borders. A directed graph is constructed from the straightened

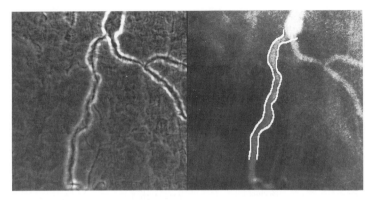

Figure 3. Conventional coronary border detection. (left) Edge image — a weighted combination of a Sobel operator and a Marr-Hildreth operator was used as an edge operator. See Figure 1 for the original angiogram. (right) Coronary borders identified using the conventional method superimposed over the original image.

edge image. A node in the directed graph corresponds to a pixel in the warped edge image. The cost associated with a node is inversely related to the edge strength of the corresponding pixel (i.e., cost is defined to be the difference between the maximum pixel value in the warped edge image and the value of each pixel). The links are defined so as to connect a node on one row of the directed graph to one of the three closest nodes on the next row. Thus, all paths through the graph contain one and only one node derived from each of the profile lines in the vessel segment of interest. This link definition ensures that all detected coronary borders are continuous in the warped image space. The node with lowest cost in the first row (greatest edge strength on perpendicular profile at proximal end of vessel segment of interest) is defined as the initial start node. The other nodes from the first row are also included as possible start nodes. The nodes on the last row of the graph are defined as goal nodes. Using these definitions for start and goal nodes, the path is not restricted to start or finish at any particular points, but is required to start and finish at the proximal and distal ends of the vessel segment of interest. Each path through the graph corresponds to a possible coronary border. The path with minimum cost is defined as corresponding to the optimal coronary border. For each vessel segment of interest, two independent searches are performed, one for the left border and one for the right border.

4.5.3. Diameter Function Calculation

After the optimal borders are identified in the straightened image space, the detected borders are mapped back into the original image space and smoothed. A diameter function depicting serial diameters along the length of the vessel is calculated and expressed in units of mm by reference to a catheter of known size. The minimal lumen diameter and the location of the minimum are automatically determined from the diameter function.

In the conventional coronary border detection method described above, coronary borders are determined using the conventional method for coronary border detection based on two-dimensional graph searching principles. This method is conventional in that it identifies the left and right coronary borders separately.

Although the method[20] was demonstrated to yield accurate borders by comparison to independent geometric (Brown-Dodge quantitative coronary arteriography) and physiological (intracoronary measures of coronary vasodilator reserve) standards and the accuracy of the method was similar in good images and in images with poor contrast or high levels of noise, experience with conventional automated methods, including those available commercially, suggests that even the most robust conventional techniques often fail to identify acceptable borders. The failure rate is especially high when these methods are routinely applied to unselected images in a clinical setting. Images with poor contrast, high noise, branching vessels, or nearby or overlapping structures present particular problems for automated techniques. Conventional automated methods for coronary border detection fail in part because they identify the left and right borders independently. Clearly, there is information contained in the position of one border that might be useful in identifying the position of the other border.

4.6. SIMULTANEOUS CORONARY BORDER DETECTION

While all existing conventional border detection algorithms independently identify the left and right coronary borders, the main principle of the simultaneous border detection is that it takes into consideration mutual relationships between borders.[68−71] As a result, the left and right borders are interrelated in agreement with physical reality. The developed strategy corresponds well with human approach to border detection. The basic steps in the simultaneous border detection algorithm are:

1. image preprocessing;
2. three-dimensional graph construction;
3. cost function calculation;
4. multi-stage identification of the optimal border pair; and
5. calculation of a diameter function.

Steps 1 and 5 are identical to those described in Section 4.5.

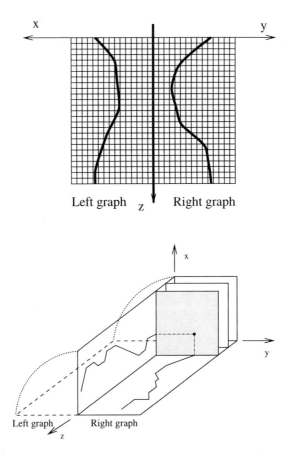

Figure 4. Three-dimensional graph construction. The top panel illustrates separate identification of the left and right borders by linking nodes in individual two-dimensional graphs corresponding to the left and right halves of the vessel segment of interest. By "rotating up" the left graph, a three-dimensional graph results in which paths correspond to pairs of coronary borders.

4.6.1. Three-dimensional Graph Construction

A major contribution of the simultaneous border detection method is the formulation of the problem of identifying both coronary borders simultaneously as a three-dimensional (3-D) graph searching problem. Shown at the top of Figure 4 are two adjacent but independent two-dimensional graphs.

Nodes in these two graphs correspond to pixels in the straightened edge image. The column of nodes separating the left graph and the right graph corresponds to the pixels on the vessel centerline. A row of nodes in the left graph corresponds to the resampled pixels along a line perpendicular to and left of the vessel centerline. If one connects nodes in the left graph together with links as shown in Figure 4, the resulting path corresponds to a possible position for the left border of the coronary artery. Similarly, linking nodes together in the right graph produces a path corresponding to a possible position of the right coronary border. In the conventional border detection method described earlier, one of the 2-D graphs is independently searched to identify the optimal left coronary border and the second 2-D graph is searched for the optimal right coronary border.

The process of constructing the three-dimensional graph can be visualized as one of rotating up the 2-D graph corresponding to the pixels left of the vessel centerline (bottom panel of Figure 4). The result is a three-dimensional array of nodes in which each node corresponds to possible positions of the left and right vessel borders for a given point along the length of the vessel. A path through the graph corresponds to a possible pair of left and right coronary borders. Nodes in the 3-D graph are referenced by their (x, y, z) coordinates. For a point along the vessel centerline defined by the z-coordinate z, a node with coordinates (x_1, y_1, z) corresponds to a left border that is x_1 pixels to the left of the centerline and a right border that is y_1 pixels to the right of the centerline.

In defining paths through the 3-D graph, it is necessary to specify a successor rule; that is, the rule for linking nodes into complete paths. Since the left border must be continuous, each parent node in the 2-D graph corresponding to the left border has three successors (left panel of Figure 5a). They correspond to a left border whose distance from the centerline decreases (successor coordinate of $(x - 1, z + 1)$), increases (successor coordinate of $(x + 1, z + 1)$), or stays the same (successor coordinate of $(x, z + 1)$) as a function of position along the centerline. A similar statement holds for the right border. In the 3-D graph, each parent node has nine successors corresponding to the possible combinations of change of positions of the left and right borders with respect to the centerline (Figure 5b). For example, the successor in the top left corner of Figure 5b corresponds to the case where the distance from the centerline of both borders has decreased. With this successor rule, all paths through the 3-D graph contain one and only one node from each "profile plane" in the 3-D graph; that is, every path contains a single node derived from each of the left and right profile lines in the vessel segment of interest. This link definition ensures that detected coronary borders are continuous in the straightened image space.

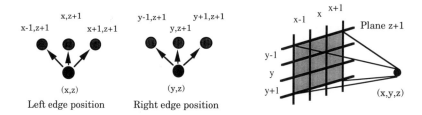

Figure 5. Successor rule in 2-D and 3-D graphs. (left) Each parent node in the separate left and right 2-D graphs has three successors. (right) Parents nodes in the 3-D graph have nine successors corresponding to the possible combinations of change in the positions of the left and right borders. (From [68], by permission of the IEEE.)

4.6.2. Identification of Optimal Border Pairs

Key aspects of the simultaneous approach for accurately identifying coronary borders are the assignment of costs to pairs of candidate borders and the identification of the optimal pair of coronary borders or lowest cost path in the 3-D graph. The cost function for a node in the 3-D graph is derived by combining the edge costs associated with the corresponding pixels on the left and right profiles in a way that allow the position of the left border to influence the position of the right border and vice versa. This strategy resembles that employed by a human observer in situations where border positions are ambiguous. In designing the cost function, the aim has been to discriminate against border pairs that are unlikely to correspond to the true vessel borders and to identify the border pair that had the greatest overall probability of matching the actual borders. The precise manner in which costs are calculated is described below.

Because of the computational complexity of the 3-D graph search, the lower bound cost adjustment is employed (see Section 4.4). It can be shown that the optimal borders detected with and without this adjustment are exactly the same. Thus, the lower bound adjustment is simply a method of substantially improving search efficiency.

As a second way to increase search efficiency, a two-stage multi-resolution approach to simultaneous border detection is implemented. In the first stage, the approximate positions of the vessel borders are identified in a low-resolution image. These approximate borders are used to guide the second-stage search by limiting the portion of the full-resolution three-dimensional graph that is searched to find the precise coronary border positions. This processing principle is known as a "coarse-to-fine" approach and is believed to be one of those incorporated in human vision.

4.6.3. Cost Function Calculation

Central to the approach to identifying optimal borders is the assignment of costs to pairs of candidate borders. The cost of a path in the 3-D graph is defined as the sum of the costs of the nodes forming the path. Costs are assigned to nodes using the following cost function:

$$C_{total}(x, y, z) = [C_s(x, y, z) + C_{pp}(x, y, z)]w(x, y) - [P_L(z) + P_R(z)]. \quad (1)$$

Each of the components of the cost function depends on the edge costs associated with image pixels. The edge costs of the left and right edge candidates located at positions x and y on profile z are inversely related to effective edge strength and are given by:

$$C_L(x, z) = \max_{x \in X, z \in Z} \{\hat{E}_L(x, z)\} - \hat{E}_L(x, z)$$

$$C_R(y, z) = \max_{y \in Y, z \in Z} \{\hat{E}_R(y, z)\} - \hat{E}_R(y, z)$$

$$(2)$$

and $\hat{E}_L(x, z)$, $\hat{E}_R(y, z)$ are straightened edge image values corrected for edge direction and are given by:

$$\hat{E}_L(x, z) = E_L(x, z) - DP_L(x, z)$$

$$\hat{E}_R(y, z) = E_R(y, z) - DP_R(y, z)$$

$$(3)$$

where $E_L(x, z)$ and $E_R(y, z)$ are straightened edge image values and $DP_L(x, z)$ and $DP_R(y, z)$ are edge direction penalties (discussed below). X and Y are sets of integers ranging from 1 to the length of the left and right halves of the vessel profiles, and Z is the set of integers ranging from 1 to the length of the vessel centerline.

The term C_s in the cost function is the sum of the edge costs for the left and right edge candidates and causes the detected borders to "follow" image positions with large gradient values. It is given by:

$$C_s(x, y, z) = C_L(x, z) + C_R(y, z). \quad (4)$$

The C_{pp} term in the cost function is useful in cases where one border has higher contrast than the opposite border and serves to cause the position of the low contrast border to be influenced by the position of the high contrast border. It is given by:

$$C_{pp}(x, y, z) = [C_L(x, z) - P_L(z)][C_R(y, z) - P_R(z)]. \qquad (5)$$

where

$$P_L(z) = \max_{x \in X, z \in Z} \{\hat{E}_L(x, z)\} - \max_{x \in X} \{\hat{E}_L(x, z)\}$$

$$(6)$$

$$P_R(z) = \max_{y \in Y, z \in Z} \{\hat{E}_R(y, z)\} - \max_{y \in Y} \{\hat{E}_R(y, z)\}$$

The $w(x, y)$ component of the cost function incorporates a model of the vessel boundary in a way that causes the positions of the left and right borders to follow certain preferred directions relative to the vessel centerline. This component has the effect of discriminating against borders that when considered as a pair are unlikely to correspond to the actual coronary borders. This is accomplished by including a weighting factor that depends on the direction by which a node is reached from its parent. The weighting factor is given by:

$$w(x, y) = 1 \quad \text{for}$$

$$(x, y) \in \{(\hat{x} - 1, \hat{y} - 1), (\hat{x}, \hat{y}), (\hat{x} + 1, \hat{y} + 1)\}$$

$$w(x, y) = \alpha \quad \text{for}$$

$$(7)$$

$$(x, y) \in \{(\hat{x} - 1, \hat{y}), (\hat{x} + 1, \hat{y}), (\hat{x}, \hat{y} - 1), (\hat{x}, \hat{y} + 1)\}$$

$$w(x, y) = \beta \quad \text{for}$$

$$(x, y) \in \{(\hat{x} - 1, \hat{y} + 1), (\hat{x} + 1, \hat{y} - 1)\}$$

where the node at coordinates (x, y) is the successor of the node at $(\hat{x}, \hat{y})$. The influence of the vessel model is determined by the values of α and β. The larger the values of α and β, the stronger is the model's influence on the detected borders.

The $P_L(z) + P_R(z)$ term in the cost function does not influence the detected border but does substantially improve search efficiency.[68]

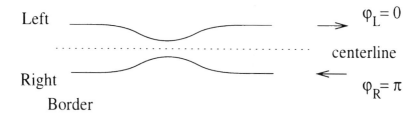

Left $\qquad \qquad \longrightarrow \quad \varphi_L = 0$

$\cdots\cdots\cdots\cdots\cdots\cdots\cdots\cdots\cdots\cdots$ centerline

Right $\qquad \qquad \longleftarrow$

Border $\qquad \qquad \varphi_R = \pi$

Figure 6. Calculation of preferred edge directions. Known edge directions for left and right borders.

4.6.4. Prior Knowledge about Local Edge Directions

To help avoid detection of vessels adjacent to the vessel of interest, knowledge about the probable direction of the actual border is incorporated into the cost function. A straightened coronary image is divided into top and bottom halves by the straightened centerline. The left and right vessel borders are located in the top and bottom halves respectively. Most but not all of the pixels along both borders have local edge directions that are horizontal and oriented from left to right for the left coronary border and right to left for the right coronary border (Figure 6). Thus, it is appropriate to discriminate in the cost function calculation against pixels whose directions are inconsistent with the known orientation of the vessel borders of interest. Local edge directions ($\varphi_L(x, z)$ for the top half or left border region and $\varphi_R(y, z)$ for the bottom half or right border region) are calculated using a 3×3 Prewitt compass operator.[62] For computational efficiency, the Prewitt operator is applied to the straightened and smoothed edge image. This operator quantitizes edge direction into one of eight possible values.

Local edge directions may depart from horizontal for a variety of reasons. Vessel borders are rarely straight, stenoses may be present, the centerline may not be positioned precisely at the lumen midline, and the images contain noise. Thus, only those pixels with edge directions outside a range of preferred directions are discriminated against. Empirically, good results are obtained by defining the preferred directions as $\varphi_L(x, z) \in [-\pi/2, \pi/2]$ for the left border and $\varphi_R(y, z) \in [\pi/2, 3\pi/2]$ for the right border. The edge direction penalty functions are calculated for the left and right borders as:

$$DP_L(x, z) = \text{penalty} \quad \text{if } \varphi_L(x, z) \notin [-\pi/2, \pi/2]$$

$$= 0 \qquad\qquad\qquad \text{otherwise}$$

$$DP_R(y, z) = \text{penalty} \quad \text{if } \varphi_R(y, z) \notin [\pi/2, 3\pi/2]$$

$$= 0 \qquad\qquad\qquad \text{otherwise} \qquad (8)$$

where *penalty* is a constant.

4.6.5. Multi-resolution and Multi-stage Border Detection

As the number of possible paths in a 3-D graph is very large, the identification of the optimal path can be very computationally demanding. For example, for a 3-D graph with xyz nodes, where z is the length in pixels of the vessel centerline, the number of possible paths is approximately 9^z. With the previously described conventional border detection method, the number of possible paths in the two two-dimensional graphs of the same size is about 3^z. Thus, the improvement in border detection accuracy achieved with simultaneous border detection is accomplished at the expense of a substantial increase in computational complexity.

To improve the speed of the algorithm, a two-stage multi-resolution border detection method has been developed. In the first stage, an estimate of the left and right coronary border positions is computed from a low-resolution edge image. The low-resolution image is produced by averaging four adjacent pixels in the full-resolution straightened edge image. Vessel boundaries identified in the low-resolution image by the simultaneous border detection method are mapped into the full-resolution image. In the second stage, those paths in the full-resolution image that are "close" to this preliminary border pair are given preference during the graph search. This is accomplished by subtracting a border preference function from each profile in the left and right halves of the straightened edge image (Figure 7).

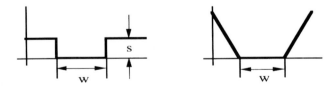

Figure 7. Border preference functions used to increase computational efficiency by constraining the search to borders close to a preliminary border pair. (From [68], by permission of the IEEE.)

Because of the inverse relationship between edge image value and edge candidate costs, this is equivalent to adding the border preference function to the edge cost profiles. This is accomplished by increasing the edge costs for nodes corresponding to pixels outside a strip of width w centered on the position of the preliminary borders. More formally, $C_L(x, z)$ and $C_R(y, z)$ are calculated as:

$$C_L(x, z) := C_L(x, z) \qquad \text{for } x_B(z) - \frac{w}{2} \leq x \leq x_B(z) + \frac{w}{2}$$

$$:= C_L(x, z) + s \qquad\qquad\qquad \text{otherwise}$$

$$C_R(y, z) := C_R(y, z) \qquad \text{for } y_B(z) - \frac{w}{2} \leq y \leq y_B(z) + \frac{w}{2}$$

$$:= C_R(y, z) + s \qquad\qquad\qquad \text{otherwise} \qquad (9)$$

where the coordinates $(x_B(z), y_B(z))$ define the approximate left and right border positions identified in the first stage, s is the cost adjustment value for pixels distant from the first-stage borders, and the symbol := represents value assignment. Other cost preference functions were also tested. The two shown in Figure 7 produced essentially the same borders. In most cases the borders produced by the multi-resolution boundary detection algorithm are exactly the same as those identified with a single phase full-resolution search process. Thus, the multi-resolution approach simply serves to increase search efficiency. Occasionally, small differences of a pixel or two in boundary location are noted.

To enhance border detection accuracy, a multi-stage border identification process has been implemented. The goal of the first stage is to reliably identify the approximate borders of the vessel segment of interest while avoiding detection of other structures. Having identified the approximate border positions, the second stage is designed to accurately localize the actual coronary borders. In the first stage, the 3-D simultaneous border detection algorithm is used to identify approximate coronary borders in half-resolution image. Since this first stage is designed in part to avoid detection of structures other than the vessel of interest, a relatively strong vessel model is used. Vessel boundaries identified in the low-resolution image are mapped into the full-resolution image and used in the second stage to guide the search for the optimal borders in the full-resolution cost image as described in the previous paragraph. A somewhat weaker vessel model (smaller values of α and β) is used in the second stage.

4.7. PERFORMANCE OF THE CONVENTIONAL AND THE SIMULTANEOUS BORDER DETECTION METHODS

To evaluate the reliability of the simultaneous border detection algorithm, the frequency was assessed with which the method failed to yield reasonable borders in complex images in which automated border detection might be expected to fail. The failure rate of the method was compared to the failure rate of a conventional border detection method. To implement multi-stage simultaneous border detection, the following parameters were used: $\alpha = 1.8$, $\beta = 2.2$ in the first stage; $\alpha = 1.2$, $\beta = 1.4$ in the second stage; a search width of $w = 8$ pixels; and cost adjustment value $s = 20$. For incorporating information about edge direction, the penalty parameter was set *penalty* $= 50$ in both stages of the search procedure.

Coronary borders were determined using the conventional method for coronary border detection based on two-dimensional graph searching principles (see Section 4.5). To allow direct comparison of the conventional and simultaneous border detection methods, the same vessel centerline and image region of interest were used for both methods.

4.7.1. Objective Measures of Border Detection Accuracy

To objectively compare coronary borders, minimal lumen diameters were calculated together with three indices of overall border configuration. For comparison with stenosis diameters determined by computer-detected methods in complex images, stenosis diameters were measured from observer-edited coronary borders. The stenosis diameter was automatically determined as the minimal lumen diameter and the stenosis location was defined as the position along the centerline of the minimal lumen diameter. For evaluation of overall border accuracy in uncomplicated images, computer-detected borders were compared by calculating the mean absolute difference and root-mean-square (rms) difference between pairs of diameter functions. A similarity index defined as the correlation coefficient between individual points on a pair of diameter functions was also calculated.

4.7.2. Assessment of Border Detection Success/Failure

An expert angiographer reviewed the digitized cine images with coronary borders detected by one of the two computer methods superimposed. For any given image, the angiographer was unaware of the border detection method employed. The angiographer identified images where automated analysis failed to produce acceptable borders. In this subjective evaluation, a border detection method was considered to have failed in a given image if: (1) a portion of the detected border corresponded to a structure other than the vessel segment of interest; (2) the presence of a sidebranch caused unacceptable distortion of the detected vessel border; or (3) the detected borders were clinically unreasonable.

4.7.3. Experimental Image Data

Effectiveness of the simultaneous border detection algorithm was evaluated in 130 "complex" coronary images. These images were selected from 439 angiograms analyzed in a previous angioplasty restenosis trial. The angiograms in this previous study were acquired before, immediately after, and 6 months following percutaneous transluminal coronary angioplasty (PTCA). As a part of this trial, all angiograms were analyzed using the conventional border detection method,[20] reviewed by an angiographer, and edited as necessary. The 130 images in which some portion of the detected borders was edited by the angiographer were selected for use in the comparison. A large number of the images in this set of 130 images contained closely parallel or overlapping vessels, adjacent structures, branching vessels, and/or were of low contrast and thus were expected to be difficult to analyze by automated methods. In addition, 43 uncomplicated images were processed that were taken from an earlier study for which the conventional border detection method gave good results in comparison to independent standards.[20]

4.7.4. Data Analysis

An experienced angiographer, who was unaware of the analysis method, visually evaluated computer-detected borders to identify those images in which the automated method failed to identify acceptable borders. Differences in analysis failure rates for simultaneous and conventional border detection were tested for significance using McNemar's test with Yates correction for continuity.[72]

Serial vessel diameters obtained from coronary borders identified by the simultaneous and conventional border detection methods were compared in 43 uncomplicated images. Conventional border detection was previously demonstrated to be accurate in these uncomplicated images by comparison to independent standards.[20] Pairs of diameter functions were compared using the mean absolute difference, rms difference, and similarity indices. Minimal lumen diameters obtained in uncomplicated images with the two border detection methods were compared using a paired t-test.

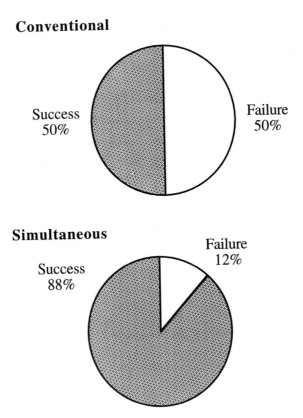

Figure 8. Failure rates of coronary border detection in complex images. Conventional border detection (above) and simultaneous border detection (below).

4.8. RESULTS

Figure 8 summarizes the results of evaluation of the reliability of simultaneous and conventional border detection in complex images. Conventional coronary border detection failed to yield acceptable borders in 65/130 or 50% of images. Simultaneous border detection failed in only 15/130 or 12% of images. In interpreting these failure rates, it should be noted that they were determined from the analysis of images that were selected because automated analysis was likely to be difficult. Simultaneous border detection was significantly more robust in the analysis of complex images than was conventional border detection ($p < 0.001$).

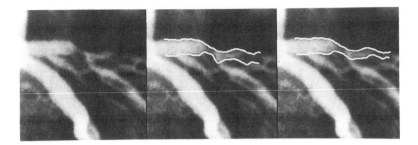

Figure 9. Border identification in a coronary artery with a closely adjacent vessel. (left) Original image. (middle) Conventional border detection incorrectly identified the vessel borders in the right end of the traced vessel, adjacent vessel border was detected instead. (right) Simultaneous border detection correctly detected both coronary borders.

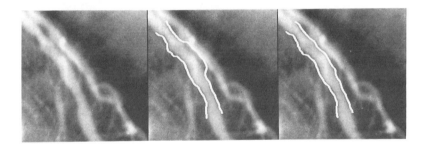

Figure 10. Border identification in a coronary artery with a closely adjacent vessel. (left) Original image. (middle) Conventional border detection was attracted to an adjacent vessel with a higher border contrast. (right) Simultaneous border detection.

Figures 9 and 10 show examples of coronary borders detected with the conventional and simultaneous border detection methods in a vessel segment with a closely adjacent vessel with higher contrast. Conventional border detection failed to identify acceptable borders of the vessel of interest while the simultaneous border detection algorithm yielded accurate borders. Example of a vessel with a stenosis located distal to a vessel branch is shown in Figure 11. Another example is given in Figure 12. Conventional border detection was not considered to have failed in this case, simultaneous border detection produced borders that were less influenced by the presence of the vessel branch.

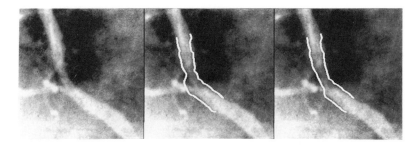

Figure 11. Border identification in a coronary artery with a lesion located distal to the bifurcation. (left) Original image. (middle) Conventional border detection failed to detect the coronary stenosis. (right) Simultaneous border detection.

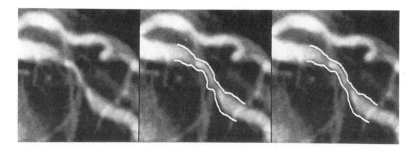

Figure 12. Border identification in a branching coronary artery. (left) Original image. (middle) Conventional border detection incorrectly traced coronary borders in the branch area. (right) Simultaneous border detection.

Stenosis diameters obtained using simultaneous border detection in complex images correlated well ($r = 0.89$, $y = 0.89x + 0.37$) with stenosis diameters derived from observer-edited borders (Figure 13a). Stenosis diameters obtained using conventional border detection correlated modestly ($r = 0.73$, $y = 0.68x + 0.84$) with stenosis diameters derived from observer-edited borders (Figure 13b). The difference in the correlation coefficients was highly significant ($p < 0.001$). Moreover, simultaneous border detection yielded a regression intercept and slope that more closely approximated zero and one respectively than did the intercept and slope obtained with conventional border detection ($p < 0.005$ for both parameters). The mean absolute difference in stenosis diameters calculated from computer-determined and observer-defined borders was 0.26 ± 0.32 mm for simultaneous border detection and 0.43 ± 0.49 mm for conventional border detection ($p < 0.001$).

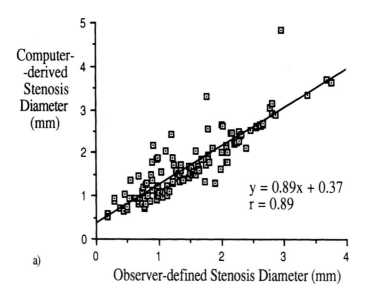

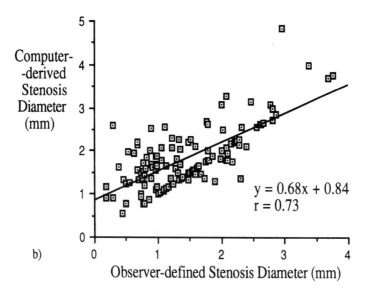

Figure 13. Comparison of computer-determined and observer-defined stenosis diameters identified in complex images. (a) Conventional border detection. (b) Simultaneous border detection. (From [70], by permission of the IEEE.)

The overall configuration of borders identified in uncomplicated images using simultaneous border detection closely approximated that obtained with conventional border detection. The average absolute difference in serial diameters along the length of the vessel was 0.09 ± 0.11 mm, the root-mean-square difference was 0.13 ± 0.16 mm, and the similarity index was 0.96 ± 0.07. Simultaneous border detection produced minimal lumen diameters in uncomplicated images that correlated well ($r = 0.98, y = 1.06x - 0.10$) with those obtained with conventional border detection. The mean difference in minimal lumen diameters was 0.01 ± 0.15 mm ($p = 0.69$). The mean absolute difference in minimal lumen diameters was 0.08 ± 0.12 mm.

4.9. COMPUTATIONAL CONSIDERATIONS

One of the challenges of simultaneous border detection was to achieve reasonable processing times compared to the conventional method. Because of substantial memory and processing requirements of the 3-D graph searching algorithm, special attention was paid to careful design of data structures. Three major data structures were employed: the straightened edge image described above, a *graph* data structure with one record for each node in the 3-D graph, and the *open_list*. The *graph* data structure was statistically allocated and consisted of a one-dimensional array of records. Each record required 13 bytes of memory and contained fields for the cost of the corresponding node, the status of the node (*not_expanded, on_open*, or *on_closed*),[62,73] a pointer to its corresponding open list element, and an offset in the *graph* structure to the record corresponding to its parent node. The open list pointer field was valid only when the status of the node was *on_open*. The *graph* data structure was "filled in" during the search process. Thus, only those records corresponding to nodes generated during the search were created. In particular, cost calculations were performed at the time nodes were generated. Records were accessed in the *graph* structure by computing an offset based on the (x, y, z) coordinates of the corresponding node.

The *open_list* data structure was a triply-linked height-balanced binary search tree.[74] As nodes were generated and placed on the open list, *open_list* records were dynamically created. Each record contained fields for the partial path cost to the node, the (x, y, z) coordinates of the corresponding node, a balance factor describing the relative heights of the left and right subtrees of the record, and pointers to the three adjacent records (i.e., parent, left and right sibling records) in the binary tree. The balance factor was used to keep the binary search tree balanced in order to maintain optimum access times to the open list. Records were inserted into the *open_list* structure so that records remained sorted according to partial path costs.

To compare computational efficiency of the simultaneous and conventional border detection algorithms, the percentage of nodes expanded (e.g., placed on the open list) during processing of a set of 43 images was measured. To determine the computational advantage of multi-resolution processing, we measured the same parameters both with and without the initial half-resolution stage used to identify a preliminary border pair.

Percentage of nodes expanded during the search was used as a computational efficiency index. The performance indices are average values obtained from 43 images with graph sizes ranging from $49 \times 49 \times 26 = 62,426$ nodes to $50 \times 50 \times 350 = 875,000$ nodes. The conventional border detection method, based on two-dimensional graph searching, expanded $85.8 \pm 9.7\%$ of the nodes in the 2-D graph to complete the border identification graph search. The simultaneous border detection method expanded $2.0 \pm 0.9\%$ of the nodes in the 3-D graph to identify borders. Although the percentage of nodes expanded in the 3-D graph was quite small compared to the percentage expanded in the 2-D graph, the 3-D graph contained a much larger number of nodes. Nonetheless, with appropriate selection of a cost function, careful attention to data structure design, incorporation of the lower bound adjustment, and use of a multi-resolution approach, computational time of a simultaneous border detection algorithm is comparable to that of the above described conventional method.[68]

The contribution of using a two-stage multi-resolution approach was also substantial. Of particular note is the six-fold improvement in worst case performance (e.g., longest graph search time) of the simultaneous border detection method that results from use of a multi-resolution approach. The graph search execution time obtained using multi-resolution processing decreased on average by a factor of 2.1 with a maximum decrease by a factor of 8.3. Execution time is a function of the size of the vessel segment of interest, vessel contrast, and complexity of the image pattern. Generally speaking, multi-resolution processing is particularly advantageous in images with branching, overlapping, or parallel vessels. The 3-D graph for such images often contains many paths with costs near the cost of the optimal path and thus increased search time is required.

4.10. RELIABILITY OF SIMULTANEOUS CORONARY BORDER DETECTION

The reliability of the simultaneous border detection method results from two key characteristics of the algorithm. The first is the use of a multi-stage strategy for identifying coronary borders that is both model and data driven. One of the limitations of model-driven image analysis procedures is that the analysis may be influenced to too great an extent by an imperfect model and thus yield inaccurate results. Giving less weight to the model resolves this problem but the analysis may fail completely in complex images where the information in the image data is insufficient to yield an accurate analysis. Thus, selection of model parameters and the relative influence to assign to the model and the image data is often a trade-off between the desire for high reliability and good accuracy. Both goals were achieved by using a two-stage analysis procedure. The first stage was intended to identify approximate coronary borders while discriminating against potential borders that were unlikely to correspond to the actual coronary borders. Having identified the approximate positions of the borders, the second stage was designed to accurately localize the coronary borders. To achieve computational efficiencies and having in mind that the first stage was not intended to identify borders with high accuracy, a low resolution edge image was used in the first stage. Because the goals of the two processing stages differed, somewhat different cost functions were employed in the two stages in order to obtain both good reliability and good accuracy. The influence of the model was greater in the first stage while the influence of the image data was greater in the second stage.

The second characteristic contributing to the reliability of the border detection method is the nature of the cost function used to define the optimal border pair. The cost function resulted from considerable experimentation and was a nonlinear combination of the edge costs associated with image pixels on the left and right vessel borders. The edge costs were related to local edge strength corrected for edge direction. The correction for edge direction was designed to help address a particularly vexing problem in the analysis of coronary angiograms — the presence of structures with high contrast adjacent to the vessel segment of interest. In effect, we took advantage of prior knowledge about the expected orientation of the border to be detected. This was accomplished by reducing the edge strength of pixels with "inappropriate" edge directions by subtracting an edge direction penalty. Prewitt compass operator was used to calculate local edge direction. Because of the influence of image noise and since the actual border orientation varies somewhat about its general direction, the edge strength was reduced only when the associated edge direction fell outside a range centered on the expected border direction. The effectiveness of this approach was determined empirically to be insensitive to the exact value of the edge direction penalty.

One method of avoiding the detection of parallel vessels is to carefully define a vessel region of interest that excludes adjacent structures. While this approach is generally effective, it may require additional operator time and/or experience and may increase inter- and intra-observer variability. This approach is unsatisfactory in the presence of branching vessels since

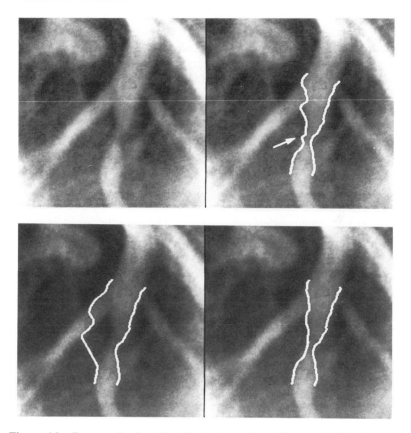

Figure 14. Coronary borders identified using region of interest (ROI) of different sizes. (top-left) Original angiographic image of a vessel segment. (top-right) Conventional coronary border detection method using a narrow ROI. Note the inaccuracy of border detection in stenosis caused by a nearby structure (depicted by an arrow). (bottom-left) Conventional method using a medium-size ROI. (bottom-right) Simultaneous coronary border detection method using a wide ROI. Borders were accurately identified even with a very wide ROI.

a variable amount of the branch vessel will always be included in the region of interest no matter how narrowly the region is defined. It has been our experience that the reliability of conventional border detection methods is very sensitive to the inclusion of adjacent structures and thus quite dependent upon the precise definition of the region of interest. Simultaneous border detection approach is quite insensitive to the care with which vessel regions of interest are defined (Figure 14).

The principal advantage of simultaneous border detection relates to its improved reliability compared to conventional methods in images where the information contained in local edge gradients is not sufficient to identify border positions. Images with very poor contrast, high levels of noise, nearby or overlapping structures, or branching vessels all present particular difficulties for conventional border detection methods that separately identify the left and right borders. While conventional analysis failed in 50% of the images, the simultaneous border detection method only failed in 12%. The reduction in failure rate was highly significant. It is worth remembering that the analyzed images were selected because they were expected to be difficult to analyze. Thus, the failure rates of both conventional and simultaneous border detection should both be less in an unselected set of images. The relative advantage of simultaneous border detection is likely to remain however since simultaneous and conventional border detection yield similar results in uncomplicated images.

4.11. CONCLUSION

A robust method for simultaneously identifying the left and right coronary borders has been described. Intuitively, it is apparent that if the position of one border is known, that information can profitably be used to identify the position of the other border. The presented strategy attempts to utilize such information to identify both borders simultaneously. This approach should be particularly useful when the location of an individual border is ambiguous in the sense that it cannot be reliably detected based upon local gradient information.

The simultaneous border detection method identifies an optimal pair of borders using a three-dimensional graph searching approach. The utilized optimization criterion (e.g., path cost) incorporates information about the global characteristics of the border pair into the detection process. It also serves to favor borders with particular characteristics and to discriminate against border pairs that are unlikely to correspond to the true borders. The implemented cost function causes a high-contrast border to more strongly influence the position of the opposite border than does a low-contrast border. Thus, a low-contrast border will tend to "follow" the opposite border if it is a high-contrast border. This behavior mimics that of a human observer who will often initially focus on locating the coronary border that can be identified with the greatest confidence and then look for the opposite border. The cost function also tends to favor pairs of borders that follow preferred directions. Thus, a border pair in which both borders approach the centerline (at the site of a stenosis for example) is judged to be more likely than one border that approaches while the other moves away from the centerline. The cost function employed in this study was the result of substantial experimentation. The principal intent in selecting a cost function was to identify the border pair that in an overall sense had the greatest probability of corresponding to the actual coronary borders.

The principal advantage of the simultaneous border detection method compared to conventional identification of individual borders relates to its improved accuracy in images in which local information contained in edge gradients is insufficient to reliably detect borders. Vessel segments with poor contrast, branching vessels, or nearby or overlapping structures often require use of global information in order to correctly identify borders. In such images, utilizing information from both borders simultaneously is advantageous. In uncomplicated images, simultaneous border detection produces borders that closely approximate those produced by conventional border detection.

Even though the shortcomings of visual assessment of coronary obstruction severity from angiograms are widely recognized, quantitative coronary angiography methods are rarely employed in routine patient care. This is due in substantial part to the fact that automated border detection methods too frequently fail to identify accurate borders, particularly in complex images. Existing border detection methods fail in part because they separately identify the left and right coronary borders. The method presented here for simultaneous identification of both coronary borders takes advantage of *a priori* clinical knowledge about border pairs. The method is highly robust and has substantial promise for enhancing the utility of quantitative coronary angiography in the routine care of patients.

4.12. ACKNOWLEDGEMENTS

This work was supported in part by the American Heart Association, Iowa Affiliate; Specialized Center of Research in Ischemic Heart Disease; National Heart, Blood, and Lung Institute; and National Institute of Health. The conventional coronary border detection and simultaneous coronary border detection methods and their results were originally published in IEEE Transactions on Medical Imaging and are reprinted with permission of the IEEE.

4.13. REFERENCES

1. Gould, K.L., 1991, *Coronary Artery Stenosis*. Elsevier, New York.
2. Skorton, D.J. and S.M. Collins, 1985, New directions in cardiac imaging. *Ann. Intern. Med.*, **102**, 795–799.
3. Stadius, M.L. and E.L. Alderman, 1990, Coronary artery revascularization. Critical need for, and consequences of, objective angiographic assessment of lesion severity. *Circulation*, **82**, 2231–2234.

4. Mancini, G.B.J., 1991, Quantitative coronary arteriographic methods in the interventional catheterization laboratory: An update and perspective. *J. Am. Coll. Cardiol.*, **17**(6), 23B–33B.

5. Zir, L.M., S.W. Miller, R.E. Dinsmore, J.P. Gilbert and J.W. Harthorne, 1976, Interobserver variability in coronary angiography. *Circulation*, **53**, 627–632.

6. Detre, K.M., E. Wright, M.L. Murphy and T. Takaro, 1975, Observer agreement in evaluating coronary angiograms. *Circulation*, **52**, 979–986.

7. De Rouen, T.A., J.A. Murray and T. Takaro, 1977, Observer agreement in evaluating coronary angiograms. *Circulation*, **55**, 324–328.

8. White, C.W., C.B. Wright, D.B. Doty, L. Hiratzka, C.L. Eastham, D.G. Harrison and M.L. Marcus, 1984, Does visual interpretation of the coronary arteriogram predict the physiologic importance of coronary stenosis? *New Engl. J. Med.*, **310**, 819–824.

9. Ross, A.M., 1990, Interpretation of coronary angiograms. *J. Am. Coll. Cardiol.*, p. 114.

10. Gould, K.L., 1992, Quantitative analysis of coronary artery restenosis after coronary angioplasty — has the rose lost its bloom? *J. Am. Coll. Cardiol.*, **19**, 946–947.

11. Marcus, M.L., D.J. Skorton, M.R. Johnson, S.M. Collins, D.G. Harrison and R.E. Kerber, 1988, The coronary arteriogram: A battered gold standard. *J. Am. Coll. Cardiol.*, **11**, 882–885.

12. Beauman, G.J. and R.A. Vogel, 1990, Accuracy of individual and panel visual interpretations of coronary arteriograms: Implications for clinical decisions. *J. Am. Coll. Cardiol.*, pp. 108–113.

13. Brown, B.G., E. Bolson, M. Frimer and H. Dodge, 1977, Quantitative coronary arteriography estimation of dimensions, hemodynamic resistance, and atheroma mass of coronary artery lesions using the arteriogram and digital computation. *Circulation*, **55**, 329–337.

14. Spears, J.R., D.P. Sandor, A. Als, M. Malagold, J.E. Markis, W. Grossman, J.R. Serur and S. Paulin, 1983, Computerized image analysis for quantitative measurement of vessel diameter from cineangiograms. *Circulation*, **68**, 453–461.

15. Reiber, J.H.C., C.J. Kooijman, C.J. Slager, J.J. Gerbrands, J.C.H. Schuurbiers, A. Den Boer, W. Wijns and P.W. Serryus, 1984, Computer assisted analysis of the severity of obstructions from coronary cineangiograms: A methodological review. *Automedica*, **5**, 219–238.

16. Kirkeeide, R.L., K.L. Gould and L. Parsel, 1986, Assessment of coronary stenoses by myocardial perfusion imaging during pharmacological coronary vasodilation. VII. validation of coronary flow reserve as a single integrated functional measure of stenosis severity reflecting all its geometric dimensions. *J. Am. Coll. Cardiol.*, **7**, 103–113.

17. Kirkeeide, R.L., P. Fung, R.W. Smalling and K.L. Gould, 1982, Automated evaluation of vessel diameter from arteriograms. In *Computers in Cardiology*, pp. 215–218, Los Alamitos, CA, IEEE.

18. Ellis, S., W. Sanders, C. Goulet, R. Miller, K.C. Cain, J. Lesperanz, M.G. Bourassa and E.L. Alderman, 1986, Optimal detection of the progression of coronary artery disease: Comparison of methods suitable for risk factor intervention trials. *Circulation*, **74**, 1235–1242.

19. Mancini, G.B.J., S.B. Simon, M.J. McGillem, M.T. Le Free, H.Z. Friedman and R.A. Vogel, 1987, Automated quantitative coronary angiography: Morphologic and physiologic validation *in vivo* of a rapid digital angiographic method. *Circulation*, **75**, 452–460.

20. Fleagle, S.R., M.R. Johnson, C.J. Wilbricht, D.J. Skorton, R.F. Wilson, C.W. White, M.L. Marcus and S.M. Collins, 1989, Automated analysis of coronary arterial morphology in cineangiograms: Geometric and physiologic validation in humans. *IEEE Trans. Med. Imaging*, **8**, 387–400.

21. Selzer, R.H., C. Hagerty, S.P. Azen, M. Siebes, P. Lee, A. Shircore and D.H. Blankenhorn, 1989, Precision and reproducibility of quantitative coronary angiography with applications to controlled clinical trials. *J. Clin. Invest.*, **83**, 520–526.

22. Eichel, P.H., E.J. Delp, K. Koral and A.J. Buda, 1988, Method for a fully automatic definition of coronary arterial edges from cineangiograms. *IEEE Trans. Med. Imaging*, **7**, 313–320.

23. Wong, W., R.L. Kirkeeide and K.L. Gould, 1986, Computer applications in angiography. In S.M. Collins and D.J. Skorton, editors, *Cardiac Imaging and Image Processing*, pp. 206–238. McGraw Hill, New York.

24. Reiber, J.H.C., P.W. Serruys and J.D. Barth, 1991, Quantitative coronary angiography. In M.L. Marcus, H.R. Schelbert, D.J. Skorton and G.L. Wolf, editors, *Cardiac Imaging*, pp. 211–280. W.B. Saunders, Philadelphia.

25. Buchi, M., O.M. Hess, R.L. Kirkeeide, T. Suter, M. Muser, H.P. Osenberg, P. Niederer, M. Anliker, K.L. Gould and H.P. Krayenbuhl, 1990, Validation of a new automatic system for biplane coronary arteriography. *Int. J. Cardiac Imag.*, **5**, 93–103.

26. Gould, K.L., R.A. Goldstein, N.A. Mullani, R.L. Kirkeeide, W. Wong, T.J. Tewson, M.S. Berridge, L.A. Bolomey, R.K. Hartz, R.W. Smalling, F. Fuentes and A. Nishikawa, 1986, Noninvasive assessment of coronary stenoses by myocardial perfusion imaging during pharmacologic coronary vasodilation. VIII. Clinical feasibility of positron cardiac imaging without a cyclotron using generator-produced rubidium-82. *J. Am. Coll. Cardiol.*, **7**, 775–789.

27. Topol, E.J., R.M. Califf, M. Vandormael, C.L. Grines, B.S. Gearge, M.L. Sanz, T. Wall, M. O'Brien, M. Swaiger, F.V. Aguirre, S. Young, J.J. Popma, K.N. Sigmon, K.L. Lee, S.G. Ellis and the TIMI-6 Study Group, 1992, A randomized trial of late reperfusion therapy for acute myocardial infarction. *Circulation*, **85**, 2090–2099.

28. de Feyter, P.J., P.W. Serruys, M.J. Davies, P. Richardson, J. Lubsen and M.F. Oliver, 1991, Quantitative coronary angiography to measure progression and regression of coronary atherosclerosis. *Circulation*, **84**, 412–423.

29. Jost, S., J. Deckers, W. Rafflenbeul, H. Hecker, U. Nellessen, B. Wiese, P.G. Hugenholtz, R.R. Lichtlen and the INTACT Study Group, 1990, Features of the angiographic evaluation of the INTACT study. *Cardiovasc. Drugs Ther.*, **4**, 1037–1046.

30. Ornisch, D., S.E. Brown, L.E. Scherwitz, J.H. Billings, W.T. Armstrong, T.A. Ports, S.M. McLanakan, R.L. Kirkeeide, R.J. Brand and K.L. Gould, 1990, Can lifestyle changes reverse coronary heart disease? The lifestyle heart trial. *Lancet*, **336**, 129–133.

31. Goldberg, R.K., N.S. Kleiman, S.T. Minor, J. Abukhalil and A.E. Raizner, 1990, Comparison of quantitative coronary angiography to visual estimates of lesion severity pre- and post-PTCA. *Am. Heart J.*, **119**, 178–184.

32. Fleming, R.W., R.C. Kirkeeide, R.W. Smalling and K.L. Gould, 1991, Patterns in visual interpretation of coronary arteriograms as detected by quantitative coronary arteriography. *J. Am. Coll. Cardiol.*, **18**, 945–951.

33. Reiber, J.H.C., 1991, An overview of coronary quantitation techniques as of 1989. In J.H.C. Reiber and P.W. Serruys, editors, *Quantitative Coronary Angiography 1991*, pp. 55–132. Kluwer Academic Publishers, Dordrecht, The Netherlands.

34. Johnson, M.R., D.J. Skorton, E.E. Ericksen, S.R. Fleagle, R.F. Wilson, L.F. Hiratzka, C.W. White, M.L. Marcus and S.M. Collins, 1988, Videodensitometric analysis of coronary stenoses: *In vivo* geometric and physiologic validation in humans. *Invest. Radiol.*, **23**, 891–898.

35. Nichols, A.B., C.F.O. Gabriele, Jr. J.J. Fenoglio and P.D. Esser, 1984, Quantification of relative arterial stenosis by cinevideodensitometric analysis of coronary arteriograms. *Circulation*, **69**, 512–522.

36. Wiesel, J., A.M. Grunwald, C. Tobiasz, B. Robin and M.M. Bodenheimer, 1986, Quantitation of absolute area of a coronary arterial stenosis: Experimental validation with a preparation *in vivo*. *Circulation*, **74**, 1099–1106.

37. Simmons, M.A., A.D. Muskett, R.A. Kruger, S.C. Klausner, N.A. Burton and J.A. Nelson, 1988, Quantitative digital subtraction coronary angiography using videodensitometry: An *in vivo* analysis. *Invest. Radiol.*, **23**, 98–106.

38. Whiting, J.S., J.M. Pfaff and N.L. Eigler, 1991, Advantages and limitations of videodensitometry in quantitative coronary angiography. In J.H.C. Reiber and P.W. Serryus, editors, *Quantitative Coronary Angiography 1991*, pp. 55–132. Kluwer Academic Publishers, Dordrecht, The Netherlands.

39. Herrold, E.M., H.L. Goldberg, J.S. Borer, K. Wong and J.W. Moses, 1990, Relative insensitivity of densitometric stenosis measurement to lumen edge detection. *J. Am. Coll. Cardiol.*, **15**, 1570–1577.

40. Johnson, M.R., G.P. Brayden, E.E. Ericksen, S.M. Collins, D.J. Skorton, D.G. Harrison, M.L. Marcus and C.W. White, 1986, Changes in coronary lumen cross-sectional area in the six months after angioplasty: A quantitative analysis of the variable response to percutaneous transluminal angioplasty. *Circulation*, **73**, 467–475.

41. Serruys, P.W., J.H.C. Reiber, W. Wijns, M. Brand, C.J. Kooijman, H.J. ten Katen and P.G. Hugenholtz, 1984, Assessment of percutaneous transluminal coronary angioplasty by quantitative coronary arteriography: Diameter versus densitometric area measurements. *Am. J. Cardiol.*, **54**, 482–488.

42. Suilen, P.A.C., N. Guggenheim, P.A. Dorsaz, F. Chappuis and W. Rutishauser, 1992, Morphometry versus densitometry — a comparison by use of casts of human coronary arteries. *Int. J. Cardiac Imag.*, **8**, 121–130.

43. Mancini, G.B.J., 1991, Applications of digital angiography to the coronary circulation. In M.L. Marcus and D.J. Skorton, editors, *Cardiac Imaging: Principles and Practice*, pp. 310–347. W.B. Saunders, Philadelphia.

44. Waters, D., J. Lesperance, T.E. Craven, G. Hudon and L.D. Gillam, 1993, Advantages and limitations of serial coronary arteriography for the assessment of progression and regression of coronary atherosclerosis. Implications for clinical trials. *Circulation*, **87**, II38–II47.

45. Sanz, M.L., G.B.J. Mancini, M.T. LeFree, J.K. Mickelson, M.R. Starling, R.A. Vogel and E.J. Topol, 1987, Variability of quantitative digital subtraction coronary angiography before and after percutaneous transluminal coronary angioplasty. *Am. J. Cardiol.*, **60**, 55–60.

46. Katritsis, D., D.A. Lythall, M.H. Anderson, I.C. Cooper and M.M. Webb-Peploe, 1988, Assessment of coronary angioplasty by an automated digital angiographic method. *Am. Heart J.*, **116**, 1181–1187.

47. Slager, J.C.J., D. Keane, D.P. Foley, A. den Boer, P.A. Doriot and P.W. Serruys, 1994, Quantification of intracoronary videodensitometry: Validation study using fluid filling of human coronary casts. *Cathet. Cardiovasc. Diagn.*, **33**, 89–95.

48. Brown, G., J.J. Albers, L.D. Fisher, S.M. Schaffer, J. Lin, C. Kaplan, X. Zhao, B.D. Bisson, V.F. Fitzpatrick and H.T. Dodge, 1990, Regression of coronary artery disease as a result of intensive lipid-lowering therapy in men with high levels of Apolipoprotein B. *N. Engl. J. Med.*, **323**, 1289–1298.

49. Gould, K.L., K.O. Kelley and E.L. Bolson, 1982, Experimental validation of quantitative coronary arteriography for determining pressure-flow characteristics of coronary stenosis. *Circulation*, **66**, 930–937.

50. Harrison, D.G., C.W. White, L.F. Hiratzka, D.B. Doty, D.H. Barnes, C.L. Eastham and M.L. Marcus, 1984, The value of lesion cross-sectional area determined by quantitative coronary angiography in assessing the physiologic significance of proximal left anterior descending coronary arterial stenoses. *Circulation*, **69**, 1111–1119.

51. Le Free, M.T., S.B. Simon, G.B.J. Mancini and R.A. Vogel, 1986, Digital angiographic assessment of coronary arterial geometric diameter and videodensitometric cross-sectional area. In *Proc SPIE*, **626**, pp. 334–341, SPIE.

52. Pope, D.L., R.E. van Bree and D.L. Parker, 1988, Automated edge detection in the analysis of cardiac function and coronary anatomy. In G.B.J. Mancini, editor, *Clinical Applications of Cardiac Angiography*, pp. 55–86. Raven Press, New York.

53. van der Zwet, P.M.J. and J.H.C. Reiber, 1992, A new algorithm to detect irregular coronary boundaries: The gradient field transform. In *Computers in Cardiology*, pp. 107–110, Los Alamitos, CA, IEEE.

54. Mortensen, E., B. Morse, W. Barrett and J. Udupa, 1992, Adaptive boundary detection using 'live-wire' two-dimensional dynamic programming. In *Computers in Cardiology*, pp. 635–638, Los Alamitos, CA, IEEE Computer Society Press.

55. Serruys, P.W., H.E. Luijten, K.J. Beatt, R. Geuskens, P.J. de Feyter, M. van den Brand, J.H.C. Reiber, H.J. ten Katen, G.A. van Es and P.G. Hugenholtz, 1988, Incidence of restenosis after successful coronary angioplasty: A time related phenomenon. A quantitative angiographic study in 342 consecutive patients at 1, 2, 3 and 4 months. *Circulation*, **77**, 361–371.

56. Gould, K.L., R.L. Kirkeeide and M. Buchi, 1990, Coronary flow reserve as a physiologic measure of stenosis severity. *J. Am. Coll. Cardiol.*, **15**, 459–474.

57. Fisher, L.D., M.P. Judkins, J. Lesperance, A. Cameron, P. Swaye, T. Ryan, C. Maynard, M. Bourassa, J.W. Kennedy, A. Gosselin, H. Kemp, D. Faxon, L. Wexler and K.B. Davis, 1982, Reproducibility of coronary arteriographic reading in the coronary artery surgery study (CASS). *Cathet. Cardiovasc. Diagn.*, **8**, 565–575.

58. Arnett, E.N., J.M. Isner, D.R. Redwood, K.M. Kent, W.P. Baker, H. Ackerstein and W.C. Roberts, 1979, Coronary artery narrowing in coronary heart disease: Comparison of cineangiographic and necropsy findings. *Ann. Intern. Med.*, **91**, 350–356.

59. Zijlstra, F., J. van Ommeren, J.H.C. Reiber and P.W. Serruys, 1987, Does the quantitative assessment of coronary artery dimensions predict the physiologic significance of a coronary stenosis? *Circulation*, **75**, 1154–1161.

60. Gurley, J.C., S.E. Nissen, D.C. Booth and A.N. DeMaria, 1992, Influence of operator- and patient-dependent variables on the suitability of automated quantitative coronary arteriography for routine clinical use. *J. Am. Coll. Cardiol.*, **19**, 1237–1243.

61. Boller, A., J. Lesperance, D. Revel, J. Marchand and M. Amiel, 1989, Automatic quantitative analysis of vascular stenosis: Experimental study of a digital angiography system applied to cardiology. *Arch. Mal. Coeur.*, **82**, 381–390.

62. Sonka, M., V. Hlavac and R. Boyle, 1993, *Image Processing, Analysis, and Machine Vision*. Chapman and Hall, London, New York.

63. Bellmann, R., 1957, *Dynamic Programming*. Princeton University Press, Princeton, NJ.

64. Pontriagin, L.S., 1962, *The Mathematical Theory of Optimal Processes*. Interscience, New York.

65. Pontriagin, L.S., 1990, *Optimal Control and Differential Games: Collection of Papers*. American Mathematical Society, Providence, RI.

66. Martelli, A., 1976, An application of heuristic search methods to edge and contour detection. *Comm. of the ACM*, **19**(2), 73–83.

67. Ney, H., 1992, A comparative study of two search strategies for connected word recognition: Dynamic programming and heuristic search. *IEEE Trans. Pattern Anal. and Machine Intelligence*, **14**(5), 586–595.

68. Sonka, M., C.J. Wilbricht, S.R. Fleagle, S.K. Tadikonda, M.D. Winniford and S.M. Collins, 1993, Simultaneous detection of both coronary borders. *IEEE Trans. Med. Imaging*, **12**, 588–599.

69. Sonka, M., M.D. Winniford, X. Zhang and S.M. Collins, 1994, Lumen centerline detection in complex coronary angiograms. *IEEE Trans. Biomed. Eng.*, **41**, 520–528.

70. Sonka, M., M.D. Winniford and S.M. Collins, 1995, Robust simultaneous detection of coronary borders in complex images. *IEEE Trans. Med. Imaging*, **14**(1), 151–161.

71. Sonka, M., G.K. Reddy, M.D. Winniford and S.M. Collins, 1993, Adaptive simultaneous coronary border detection: A method for accurate analysis of small diameter vessels. In *Computers in Cardiology*, pp. 109–112, Los Alamitos, CA, IEEE.

72. Zar, J.H., 1984, *Biostatistical Analysis*. Prentice Hall, Englewood Cliffs, 2nd edition.

73. Nilsson, N.J., 1971, *Problem Solving Methods in Artificial Intelligence*. McGraw Hill, New York.

74. Reingold, E.M. and W.J. Hansen, 1983, *Data Structures*. Little Brown and Company, Boston.

5 COMPUTER ANALYSIS OF INTRAVASCULAR ULTRASOUND IMAGES*

MILAN SONKA,[1,†] CHARLES R. McKAY[2] and
CLEMENS von BIRGELEN[3]

[1]*Department of Electrical and Computer Engineering,*
[2]*Department of Internal Medicine, The University of Iowa,*
Iowa City, IA 52242, USA
[3]*Thoraxcenter, Division of Cardiology,*
Erasmus University Rotterdam, The Netherlands

5.1. INTRODUCTION

While each of the existing methods for assessing coronary artery disease *in vivo* like coronary angiography, fluoroscopy, fiberoptic angioscopy, ultrafast computed tomography, magnetic resonance angiography, epicardial ultrasonography, and intravascular ultrasound has potential advantages,[1-4] only coronary angiography has found widespread clinical use. Coronary angiography produces projection images or silhouettes of the vascular lumen from the absorption of X-rays by radiopaque dye injected into the coronary tree.[5] The coronary wall and any atherosclerotic plaque that might be present are not directly visualized. Conclusions about the presence and significance of atherosclerosis are inferred from visual assessment of the

---

*Portions reprinted, with permission, from IEEE Transactions on Medical Imaging, Volume 14, December 1995. ©1995 IEEE.

†Correspondence: Milan Sonka, Department of Electrical and Computer Engineering, University of Iowa, Iowa City, Iowa, 52242. Phone: (319)-335-6052; Fax: (319)-335-6028; e-mail: milan-sonka@uiowa.edu.

reduction in vessel lumen diameter with respect to the lumen diameter of a nearby vessel segment that is presumed to be normal. The shortcomings of visual evaluation of lumen dimensions are widely recognized.[6] Even when employed in conjunction with quantitative analysis,[7,8] coronary angiography has several limitations. These include the inability to detect plaque in diffusely diseased vessels, inability to directly determine vessel wall and plaque morphology, inaccuracy in analyzing eccentric lesions, and insensitivity to changes in arterial morphology after catheter-based interventional therapy.

Intravascular ultrasound yields tomographic two-dimensional cross-sectional images of vessel wall architecture and plaque morphology. From the images obtained by intravascular ultrasound, morphometric measurements of lumen and plaque can directly be performed.[9,10] The principle underlying the measurements obtained from intravascular ultrasound images differs substantially from quantitative coronary angiography, which has traditionally been viewed as the "gold standard" in quantifying coronary artery dimensions. The main difference is that quantitative angiography does not permit direct measurement of plaque dimensions, but quantifies lumen diameter and obstruction based on the brightness and contours of the opacified silhouette of the coronary lumen, assuming a non-diseased reference segment.[11−13] This assumption, however, is frequently false and particularly in diffusely diseased coronary arteries, the obstruction can be significantly underestimated. Intravascular ultrasound measures lesion significance independently of the reference segments.[14] Post-mortem studies and early *in vivo* studies have shown that intravascular ultrasound yields important information about vessel morphology that is not obtained from angiography.

This chapter summarizes the use of intravascular ultrasound (IVUS) imaging in diagnostics and interventional treatment of coronary arteries and describes computer-aided approaches that help analyze IVUS images. It should be mentioned, however, that intravascular ultrasound is also used to image a variety of other vascular structures; iliac or femoral arteries being the most common example.

5.2. INTRAVASCULAR ULTRASOUND IMAGING

5.2.1. Intravascular Ultrasound Imaging Devices

With intravascular ultrasound, a high-frequency (20–50 MHz) ultrasound source rotates near the tip of a catheter inserted in the arterial lumen.[15] Either the piezoelectric crystal generating the ultrasound beam or a mirror deflecting the ultrasound beam is rotated. Alternatively, a stationary multi-element crystal array encircling the catheter may be employed. In the former case, the ultrasound element or the mirror is rotated by use of a long flexible shaft driven by an external motor. The lengths of the shaft and arterial path tortuosity may cause non-uniform rotation creating imaging artifacts. In the latest prototypes, the external motor has been replaced by a micromotor in the catheter tip. In multi-element ultrasound arrays, no mechanical rotation is involved and the signal is processed and multiplexed using an integrated circuit in the catheter tip. Possibility to use a central guide wire with a full 360° field of view is the main advantage of this design. In addition to the single-cross-sectional ultrasound imaging devices, prototypes of forward-looking catheters and imaging ultrasound guidewires have been reported.[15]

Intravascular ultrasound cross-sectional images directly demonstrate arterial lumen, plaque, and wall morphology. Figure 1 shows examples of two intravascular ultrasound images of a cylindrical latex phantom.[16,17] Intravascular ultrasound morphology, determined from operator-defined borders, agrees closely with quantitative histologic determination of lumen area and mural thickness[18,19] and angiographic determination of lumen size.[9,20,21]

5.2.2. Coronary Wall Morphology Imaged by Intravascular Ultrasound

Atherosclerosis is characterized by an accumulation of plaque material in the arterial wall. Figure 2 shows in schematic form the cross-sectional anatomy of a diseased coronary artery. In adults, normal coronary vessel walls (upper portion of Figure 2) have a thin intimal layer bounded by the internal elastic lamina. The media, composed of smooth muscle cells and a reticular collagen network is located between the internal and external elastic laminae and is of nearly constant thickness, typically 0.1–0.3 mm.[9,22−24] Outside the external elastic lamina is fibrous and fatty adventitia tissue. With progressive atherosclerosis (bottom portion of Figure 2), intimal cells proliferate, lipid and cholesterol accumulate, fibrosis occurs, and the wall thickens. As intimal plaque thickens, the media may thin and the internal lamina may be disrupted. Initially, eccentric plaque bulk increases the total wall thickness and locally distends the wall such that the lumen shape and diameter is maintained ("arterial wall remodeling"). As plaque continues to accumulate, the lumen is compromised, the plaque may become more concentric, and focal areas of calcification and extracellular lipid or cholesterol depositions ("lipid lake") are seen. Because these morphologic changes can be visualized by intravascular ultrasound, the appearance of intravascular ultrasound images can be complex.

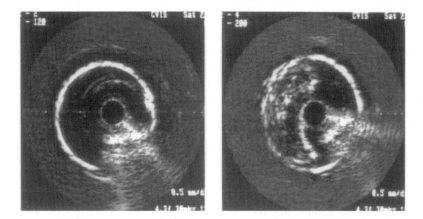

Figure 1. Intravascular ultrasound images of a cylindrical latex phantom. (left) Cross-section representing an undiseased artery. Strut artifact of the used intravascular ultrasound catheter can be seen as a noisy wedge in the 4- to 6-o'clock position. (right) Lesion cross-section. The latex wall borders and the borders between lumen and plaque are clearly visible, plaque is present in the 6- to 12-o'clock position. The strut artifact is seen in the 3- to 5-o'clock position.

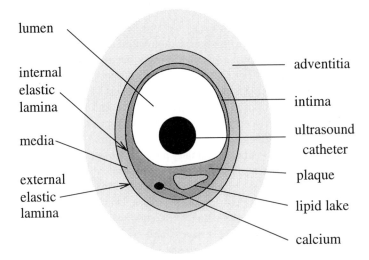

Figure 2. Schematic cross-sectional anatomy of a diseased coronary vessel (not to scale).

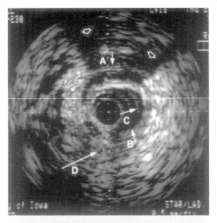

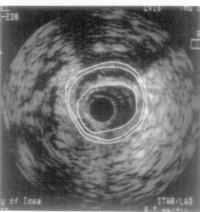

Figure 3. Intravascular ultrasound image of a diseased coronary vessel. (top) Original image with 0.5 mm calibration marks showing circumferential plaque that thickens at the 10- to 2-o'clock position. Double-echo response from the internal and external elastic laminae with intervening sonolucent media is seen at the 12-o'clock position (arrow A), and also at 10-o'clock and 5-o'clock. The interface between lumen and plaque is depicted by arrow B and is visible at 9- to 6-o'clock. The catheter near-field artifact surrounds the catheter in the middle of the image and obscures the plaque–lumen border from 6- to 9-o'clock. Arrow C shows a near-field artifact. Two wide arrows point to regions of signal attenuation caused by fibrotic plaque that is highly reflectant. The dark sonolucent region from 10- to 2-o'clock located inside the plaque is due to echo dropout distal to the fibro-calcific plaque at the lumen–plaque interface. Arrow D shows the strut and guidewire artifact. The complex plaque morphology in this vessel was confirmed with light microscopy. (bottom) Positions of external elastic lamina, internal elastic lamina, and coronary lumen defined by an observer.

The interaction of ultrasound with coronary arterial structures gives rise to typical image patterns that may be used to identify arterial wall and intramural structures within the ultrasound image (Figure 3). Intravascular ultrasound images contain both large amplitude signals from specular reflectors at the interface between structures with differing acoustic impedances together with lower amplitude signals or diffusely scattered signals arising from regions of nearly uniform acoustic properties. The lumen is typically a dark echo-free region adjacent to the imaging catheter. The lumen-intima interface constitutes a large acoustic impedance mismatch and produces specular reflections.[23] The internal and external elastic laminae enclose the sonolucent media and produce acoustic impedance mismatches. There is an ongoing discussion about what exactly causes the ultrasound echo responses. Additionally, the internal elastic lamina often partially disappears in diseased coronary vessels. The layers typically give rise to a double-echo pattern showing a circumferentially-oriented parallel bright–dark–bright echo pattern[25] (arrow A in Figure 3a). The echo-dense responses are from the interfaces of the fibro-elastic internal and external elastic laminae and the homogeneous echo-free media layer. The fibrous adventitia further demarcates the outer wall with abrupt increases in echo-density which parallel the double-echo responses from the laminae and media. With coronary artery disease, the intima thickens and is identified as the echogenic region between the lumen interface and the sonolucent media (arrow B in Figure 3a). The ultrasonic appearance of atherosclerotic plaque depends on its composition.[25] Fibromuscular lesions appear as echoes of intermediate intensity attached to the intima. Dense fibrous lesions appear as bright echoes. Calcium deposits also give rise to high intensity echoes. Lipid deposits within a lesion are hypoechoic. Analysis of intravascular ultrasound images can be complicated by focal or radial echo patterns which are generated by local changes in plaque density. For example, regions of substantially attenuated signal intensity (two wide arrows in Figure 3a) may be caused by highly echo-reflectant fibrous plaque or calcium deposits which produce acoustic shadowing.

The presence of a variety of artifacts can render the interpretation of intravascular images difficult. Blood speckle and near-field artifacts can be identified by observing the real-time video. As the catheter is pulled back, the artifacts persist while the wall morphology changes. A bright near-field "halo" adjacent to the black circle depicting the catheter's position results from ultrasound reflections from the catheter itself (arrow C in Figure 3a). These artifacts and geometric distortion due to an eccentric or angulated catheter position within the vessel may prevent visualization of the double-echo pattern from the media–laminae interfaces. In second generation catheters, a strut or guidewire artifact across the imaging plane obscures (or distorts) mural details in portions of the arterial wall (arrow D in Figure 3a).

5.3. CLINICAL IMPORTANCE OF INTRAVASCULAR ULTRASOUND IMAGING

Intravascular ultrasound imaging yields morphologic information complementary to contrast angiography. There is substantial enthusiasm in the clinical community for using this emerging imaging method to overcome the shortcomings of angiography and for guiding catheter-based interventions.[26–29] Intravascular ultrasound is capable of providing cross-sectional images of the coronary arteries and visualizing the structural[9,30–33] and functional pathology[34,35] of the coronary artery lumen and vessel wall. Plaque eccentricity, lipids, and calcification can be determined.[36] Mechanisms of plaque dilatation, recoil, and dissection after catheter-based intervention can be studied.[29] Ongoing clinical trials have presented preliminary data showing that immediately after angioplasty, intravascular ultrasound determination of minimum lumen diameter and plaque area as a percentage of total arterial cross-sectional area are predictors of restenosis within 6 months after the interventional therapy.[37]

5.3.1. Measurements of Plaque Dimensions

Intravascular ultrasound enables the quantitative study of the extent of coronary atherosclerosis. The important landmark study of Glagov et al.[38] demonstrated vessel wall remodeling — a compensatory enlargement of the vessel wall in response to progressive atherosclerosis, accommodating the increasing atherosclerotic burden up to 40% of the cross-sectional reference area. The results of Glagov's study highlight the importance of direct visualization and measurement of plaque dimensions, provided by intravascular ultrasound. Comparing histology and angiograms in coronary arteries of postmortem human hearts, Stiel et al. confirmed that the compensatory enlargement of atherosclerotic coronary arteries results in a significant angiographic underestimation of the extent of atherosclerosis during early stages of coronary artery disease.[39] In 1987, McPherson et al. demonstrated the unique capabilities of epicardial high-frequency ultrasound imaging, which has been a forerunner of intravascular ultrasound, in detecting coronary plaques in patients without angiographic evidence of atherosclerosis.[40] Intravascular ultrasound is indeed able to detect atherosclerosis in angiographically normal vessels.[41] St. Goar et al. studied the coronary arteries in cardiac transplant recipients using intravascular ultrasound. In the majority of patients who were studied one or more years after transplantation, an intimal thickening could be demonstrated that was not visible on the angiograms.[32] During the early phases, atherosclerosis can frequently be found by intravascular ultrasound at the site of a focal vasospasm,[35] which demonstrates the significant sensitivity of this technique.

Echocardiographic confirmation of the compensatory enlargement of coronary arteries during the progression of atherosclerosis was first performed intraoperatively, using high-frequency epicardial echocardiography.[42] Thereafter the mechanism could be demonstrated by intravascular ultrasound in coronary[30,43,44] and in femoral arteries.[45] However, intravascular ultrasound offers not only an ideal way of evaluating the dimensions of atherosclerotic arteries at a point in time,[28] but can also be used for serial studies, for instance in trials assessing the progression/regression of coronary atherosclerosis.[46,47] Opposite to quantitative coronary angiography, intravascular ultrasound measures dimensions independently of the reference segment disease which is likely to be involved in the process of progression or regression.

5.3.2. Lesion Calcification

5.3.2.1. Detection of lesion calcification

Identification of calcific lesions is important. Calcium appears to stabilize a non-treated plaque and protect patients against unstable clinical syndromes.[31] However, following directional coronary atherectomy, a higher incidence of complications and a smaller amount of retrievable material can be observed in the presence of diffuse subendothelial calcification[48] (Figure 4). The angiographic assessment of 400 lesions, reported by Ellis *et al.*, demonstrated an independent correlation of target lesion calcium with adverse outcome after directional coronary atherectomy.[49] Mintz *et al.* reported that coherent calcific deposits in the target lesion were discovered in 75% of patients examined by intravascular ultrasound before or after various catheter-based interventions, however, calcium confirmed by ultrasound could be detected in less than 50% of the patients during angiography.[50] Another study reported that target lesion calcification was detected by intravascular ultrasound in 83% whereas calcium was seen in only 14% of the lesions by angiography.[51] These studies demonstrate that intravascular ultrasound is much more sensitive than angiography in detecting calcium. Only visualization of accumulated microcalcifications by intravascular ultrasound appears to be limited,[52] reflecting the limited lateral resolution of the current intravascular ultrasound transducers.[53]

5.3.2.2. Relation of dissections to calcium deposits

Dissections are commonly accepted as an operative mechanism of balloon angioplasty.[54,55] However, larger dissections can cause acute vessel closure, and when confirmed by intravascular ultrasound, dissections correlate with an increased risk of subsequent adverse events after angiographically successful

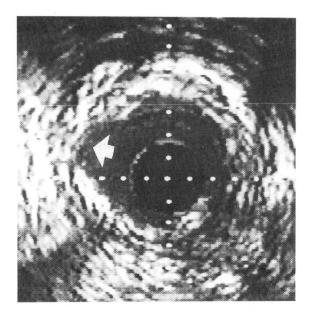

Figure 4. Cross-sectional intracoronary ultrasound image showing a cut in the vessel wall (arrowhead) resulting from the application of a directional atherectomy device. The cut is located next to a deposit of superficial calcium, obscuring the underlying vessel wall in its echo shade. A larger part of the arterial wall is obscured by another arc of deep calcium.

coronary artery interventions.[56] Fitzgerald *et al.* examined peripheral and coronary arteries of 41 patients *in vivo* after balloon angioplasty and demonstrated that in 87% of the cases, dissections were adjacent to a calcific portion of the vessel wall.[23] Furthermore, an increased incidence, depth, and circumferential extension of dissections after balloon dilatation was found in calcific segments of atherosclerotic plaques.[23,53,57] Results of these studies suggest that localized calcium deposits play a significant role in promoting the incidence of dissections.

5.3.3. Role of Intravascular Ultrasound Analysis in Pre-interventional Decision-making

Intravascular ultrasound findings frequently give rise to a modification of treatment strategy. Mintz *et al.* reported that intravascular ultrasound examination of 313 target lesions resulted in a change in therapy in 124 cases that corresponds to almost 40%.[58] In particular, lesion calcification and eccentricity were reasons for changing or selecting specific interventional devices. Generally, eccentric lesions without evidence of superficial calcium were treated with directional atherectomy, while in superficially calcified plaques rotational atherectomy or eximer laser angioplasty were performed.[58] Rotational atherectomy is particularly suitable for the treatment of superficially calcified, diffusely diseased coronary arteries, since the device ablates and pulverizes non-compliant plaque material by high-frequency rotation of a diamond-coated burr, resulting in a relatively circular and smooth shape of the coronary lumen.[59] It may be used as a stand-alone procedure but is frequently used as a primary device followed by adjunctive balloon angioplasty or directional atherectomy.[60] Thus, lesion eccentricity and the presence or absence of calcium and its superficial or deep location in the atherosclerotic plaque demonstrated by intravascular ultrasound imaging have major implications in the choice of an interventional device.

5.3.3.1. Balloon angioplasty

Serial intravascular ultrasound studies performed before and after balloon angioplasty have helped to identify the operative mechanisms of this device. In coronary and peripheral vessels *in vitro* and *in vivo*, vessel wall stretching, plaque rupture and dissection, and to some extent plaque compression were confirmed to reflect the principal operative mechanisms of balloon angioplasty.[61-64] The acute lumen gain and possible complications of a procedure such as large dissections with threatening vessel closure can be studied by intravascular ultrasound. Dissections of the coronary plaque are commonly found after balloon angioplasty,[28] but even complex dissections, frequently not detected by angiography, can be demonstrated by intravascular ultrasound.[56,57,65,66] Recently the diagnosis of a pseudoaneurysm formation following balloon angioplasty was made using intravascular ultrasound.[67] A new catheter combining ultrasound imaging and balloon angioplasty has been developed and preliminary experience with this device has demonstrated its feasibility and usefulness.[68-70] The device can be utilized to obtain additional qualitative and quantitative information about vessel lumen and wall before and after an intervention. Intravascular imaging through the angioplasty balloon permits direct examination of the vessel wall morphology and furthermore acute recoil can be evaluated immediately. The combination of a diagnostic and a therapeutic device may reduce the time required for the exchange of catheters in separate ultrasound examinations and minimize the small risk of inducing or aggravating vessel wall injury during repeated insertions of the catheters. In coronary stenting this combined approach may facilitate stent implantation and expansion and reduce the risk of stent strut damage.[71]

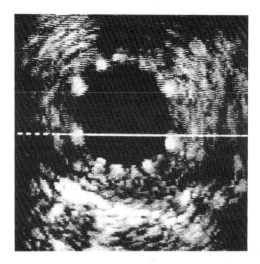

Figure 5. Well deployed Wallstent. The brightness of the echo-reflective struts allows to distinguish between the stent and the artery wall. A circular stent configuration and a good apposition to the vessel wall are demonstrated.

5.3.3.2. Coronary stenting

In acute or chronic dissection, intravascular ultrasound imaging helps to distinguish between true and false lumen and thus increase the safety of the stenting procedure.[72,73] The struts of the metal stents are echo-reflective and well visualized (Figure 5). After elective coronary stenting, Laskey *et al.* found substantial improvement of angiography-related parameters, but less favorable outcome resulted from the intravascular ultrasound examination. This emphasizes the benefit of routine ultrasound studies during the implantation of coronary stents.[74] Furthermore, information concerning a significant disease of the reference segments can only be provided by intravascular ultrasound, and thus used to control the deployment and expansion of the stent.

The major criteria of the quality of stent deployment are considered to be lumen symmetry, stent apposition to the vessel wall and the absence of a residual lumen narrowing inside the stent. Detection of a moderate residual stenosis inside the stented coronary segment by angiography is difficult. Unfortunately, such an intra-stent stenosis carries a higher chance of turbulent blood flow which can result in the accumulation of thrombus inside the stent and finally increase the risk of stent thrombosis and restenosis. The optimization of stent deployment based on the utilization of imaging and morphometric measurements by intravascular ultrasound, however, virtually eliminates the risk of acute or subacute stent thrombosis.[75] As a consequence, coronary stenting can be performed without anticoagulation.[76] The large single-center experience of Colombo et al. with intravascular ultrasound guided stenting has demonstrated an evident inadequacy of angiographically guided stenting. In order to achieve improved stent apposition, higher balloon-to-artery ratios and higher balloon inflation pressures are advocated. Ongoing multicenter studies are required to establish whether this concept without ultrasound guidance is sufficient to achieve results comparable to the outcome after ultrasound guided stenting.[77] A new mechanically rotated intravascular ultrasound guidewire[78] that can be passed centrally through the lumen of the stent delivery balloon represents a concept with the inherent potential to minimize the time required for ultrasound imaging and the risk of strut damage. The ultrasound guidewire may increase the accuracy of stent placement and may be particularly beneficial in the implantation of multiple stents.

5.3.3.3. *Directional coronary atherectomy*

Directional coronary atherectomy is particularly efficient when it is applied to "soft", eccentric plaques without superficial calcium in proximal or mid-coronary segments.[49,58,79] Popma et al. studied 57 patients after directional atherectomy using intravascular ultrasound and found that the amount of residual plaque mass remained significantly higher in lesions with an arc of calcium larger than $90°$.[80] Intravascular ultrasound is clinically useful in guiding the device since it demonstrates plaque composition and provides more reliable information about plaque eccentricity[29,48] in contrast to angiography. Ultrasound guidance facilitates the optimization of plaque removal (Figure 4) and minimizes the trauma to the non-diseased vessel wall, which appear to be important factors in the process of restenosis.[81] A prototype device combining ultrasound imaging and directional atherectomy provides images from the aperture of the atherectomy catheter.[82] This approach allows the adjustment of the orientation of the cutter, scanning the plaque portion before the excision, and thus improving the procedural result. Ultrasound imaging can be performed repeatedly when the housing of a conventional atherectome has to be emptied of accumulated samples. The ultrasound examination pre- and post-intervention provides additional information suggesting that the operative mechanism is mainly based on plaque removal but also to a certain extent on the vessel stretch.[62,64] Suneja et al. found that "plaque compression" accounts for 50% of the enlargement of lumen area, however, this finding seems to reflect the problem of pre-/post-studies which consider only changes at the site of the minimal luminal area,[83] a limitation which can only be overcome by quantification with three-dimensional ultrasound.[84,85]

5.4. AUTOMATED ANALYSIS OF INTRAVASCULAR ULTRASOUND IMAGES

To date, quantitative studies of coronary atherosclerosis have nearly always relied on manual measurements of arterial structure dimensions and manual tracing of lumen and wall borders. While a number of studies demonstrate that experienced observers can identify plaque and wall borders in intravascular ultrasound images that agree with histology and angiography,[3,26] the utility of analysis approaches relying upon manual border identification is limited by the need for observers with substantial experience and by the tedious nature of manual tracing. Recently, a number of groups have begun to develop computer-based methods for identifying lumen and wall borders.[17,50,86−88] The most experience has been gained with computer methods that are based on image intensity thresholding. These methods classify each image pixel as belonging to lumen or vessel wall and generally are unable to distinguish between plaque, intima, media, and adventitia. Very little data demonstrating the accuracy of such techniques have been reported.[89] Given the commonly recognized limitations of thresholding approaches to segmentation, it is unlikely that such approaches will be widely adopted for quantitative analysis of lumen and wall morphology from intravascular ultrasound images.

Development of methods for automated identification of lumen and mural structures has been limited in the past by the relatively poor quality of intravascular ultrasound images. Even with the recent substantial improvements in imaging catheters and signal processing hardware, accurate and robust segmentation of intravascular ultrasound images presents a very challenging problem. Studies correlating *in vitro* and *in vivo* intravascular ultrasound measurements with histology and angiography suggest that experienced observers can identify important luminal and mural structures. These studies suggest that when combined with appropriate *a priori* knowledge or context, the information necessary to perform such identification is present in the image data.

5.4.1. Approaches to Single-frame IVUS Image Analysis

Currently, visual identification of arterial wall and plaque borders is most commonly used to assess disease severity from intravascular ultrasound images. Manually traced borders of vascular structures in intravascular ultrasound images are typically used to calculate lumen and plaque cross-sectional areas to distinguish critical and non-critical lesions,[28,90] assess and classify the morphologic effects of percutaneous coronary angioplasty,[65] and compute arterial biomechanical properties.[91,92] The ability of experienced observers to integrate information from real-time image sequences and to apply *a priori* knowledge of arterial morphology are crucial determinants of the accuracy of visual border detection. A number of *in vitro* and *in vivo* studies have demonstrated the accuracy of visual border detection in intravascular ultrasound images by comparison to quantitative histopathology[3,19,22,25,65,93] and to coronary angiography.[21] The intra- and inter-observer reproducibility of lumen area and wall thickness measurements with intravascular ultrasound are good with mean percent difference between repeated determinations by the same observer of $2 \pm 9\%$ for lumen cross-sectional areas and $3.6 \pm 18\%$ for wall thicknesses, and between measurements by two observers of $1.8 \pm 15\%$ for lumen areas and $12 \pm 15\%$ for wall thicknesses.[22] While observers can manually identify accurate borders in individual intravascular ultrasound images, quantitative analysis of three-dimensional or dynamic arterial morphology based on manual tracing is impractical.

Automated or semi-automated image segmentation methods using image intensity thresholding to distinguish among vessel lumen, wall, and surrounding tissue have been employed to identify vessel lumen and to produce three-dimensional renderings of vessel geometry.[50,86,94] Vessel wall detected by these methods typically includes plaque, intima, media, and adventitia with no or limited ability to distinguish between them. Rosenfield and associates consider a voxel as part of the vessel wall if its intensity lies between minimum and maximum threshold values specified by an operator.[87,94] Threshold selection plays a crucial role in the analysis. An interactively-defined region of interest bounded by an inner and outer circle is provided by the operator and used to enclose the arterial wall and exclude the catheter and the associated ring-down artifact. Measurements of lumen area obtained with this method have been validated in comparison to quantitative angiography in an atherosclerotic swine model.[89] A similar approach was reported by Mintz and colleagues.[50] To avoid image thresholding difficulties arising from the presence of artifacts inside the vessel lumen and outside the vessel wall, they manually define regions of interest to only include arterial structures between adventitia and intima. The limitations of thresholding using fixed thresholds as a segmentation method are widely recognized in the medical imaging community. Even very careful region of interest selection does not obviate these problems. Nevertheless, substantial improvements in the utility of threshold-based segmentation can be expected with improvements in intravascular image quality.

Much effort is currently being devoted to development of blood backscatter-based techniques to clean-up the noise from the imaged vessel lumen.[15] It is a well-known observation that arterial walls tend to be represented by a more stable echo signal while the blood echo signal in the lumen is changing rapidly. The general idea of lumen image improvements is based on minimization of the blood scattering noise either by temporal averaging or sequential subtraction of image intensities in consecutive image frames,[95] or averaging of the power spectrum of RF signals from scattered ultrasound.[96−98] Texture properties of specular ultrasound signals are sometimes utilized to improve image segmentation in a variety of ultrasound image data.[99−103]

An intravascular ultrasound border detection approach which identifies wall and plaque borders that uses simulated annealing was reported by Herrington *et al.*[88] In their approach, an operator interactively identifies an approximate border and a resampled image is formed using the approximate border to define a region of interest. An edge operator was applied to the resampled image and the closed boundary that represented the best compromise between identifying a smooth boundary and minimizing the sum of the inverted edge strengths along the boundary was determined. Using this procedure, borders between blood and plaque or between media and adventitia may be individually identified. Dhawale *et al.* use interactively-defined boundary points to guide a dynamic search for the border between media and adventitia and the border between blood and plaque.[104]

We have previously reported an approach using a heuristic graph search for identifying external and internal laminae and plaque borders.[17] This method used an adaptive model-based approach in which the strength of the model varied around the vessel circumference as a function of local image quality. The method was validated in two distensible phantoms, each of which was imaged under several pressure conditions. Lumen cross-sectional areas correlated very well with distending pressure in both phantoms. Although this method yielded promising results and important insights in phantoms, it did not incorporate sufficient *a priori* information to perform well in more realistic imaging situations.

No fully automated method for detection of coronary wall and plaque borders in intravascular ultrasound images has been published to date. Intravascular ultrasound images are quite noisy and often contain catheter and other artifacts. Without contextual information from image frames adjacent in space and time, single-frame intravascular images are difficult to analyze even for the most experienced humans. To be successful, automated methods need to incorporate substantial *a priori* knowledge about ultrasound imaging physics and arterial anatomy. The ability to use information from temporally and spatially adjacent images could also prove advantageous.

5.4.2. Knowledge-based Approach to Coronary Wall and Plaque Border Detection

The following method for automated segmentation of intravascular ultrasound images developed at the University of Iowa uses global image
information and heuristic graph searching[5,105] to identify wall and plaque
borders. A priori knowledge of coronary artery anatomy and ultrasound
image characteristics were incorporated into the method for intravascular
ultrasound border detection.

The method has two key characteristics. First, it uses a graph searching
border detection approach that identifies a border that is optimal in a global
sense. This approach is particularly advantageous in images where local edge
gradients are insufficient to reliably identify border positions. Second, the
method incorporates a priori information of a variety of types into the border
detection process. In particular, to identify the position of the external elastic
lamina we search not for a connected series of pixels with large edge gradients
but for an expected double-echo edge pattern. This pattern does not rely on the
frequently reported trilayer appearance of intravascular ultrasound images of
muscular arteries. The trilayer appearance of diseased coronary vessels is
thought to correspond with sequential layers of intima and/or plaque, media,
and surrounding tissue (adventitia) and may in fact not always be present.[23]
We are instead exploiting the differences in acoustic impedance between the
elastic laminae and the surrounding tissues.[23,25]

The method searches for edge triplets representing the leading and trailing
edges of the external elastic lamina echo and the trailing edge of the internal
elastic lamina echo. It has previously been suggested that the local gradients
of trailing edges are less useful in locating borders because the trailing
edge signal is highly gain-dependent.[88] Accordingly, we do not use the
trailing edge location but rather use the existence of trailing edges inside two
windows positioned with respect to the leading edge of the external lamina
as contextual edge information. Based on the presence of this double-echo
pattern and discriminating against borders that depart too much from the
model of the preferred vessel shape, the location of the external elastic
lamina is determined. This boundary then serves to define a search region,
whose width is defined by a priori knowledge about the thickness of the
media, within which the leading edge of the internal elastic lamina echo is
determined. Lastly, the border between lumen and plaque is identified based
on the echo response from the blood–plaque interface. Thus, the identification
of all three borders is based on searching for a boundary that is globally
optimal. Consequently, it is possible to identify borders even in the presence
of missing data due, for example, to focal interruptions of the internal elastic
lamina caused by plaque.

5.4.2.1. Wall and plaque border detection algorithm

After digitization of S-VHS-recorded intravascular ultrasound images at a resolution of $512 \times 512 \times 8$ (0.03 mm/pixel), the border detection method consists of the following steps:

1. interactive definition of the region of interest;
2. edge detection and coordinate transformation of the edge image;
3. identification of the internal and external laminae and of the plaque–lumen interface;
4. mapping of all three borders back into the original image space and calculation of quantitative measures of arterial morphology.

5.4.2.2. Definition of region of interest

Due to the image ambiguities discussed in Section 5.2.2 and the problems of identifying ultrasound imaging artifacts in individual digitized frames, an operator-defined region of interest is identified prior to automated border detection. In each image, an ellipse enclosing the vessel (lumen, plaque, media and a portion of the adventitia) is manually defined by an operator. The ellipse defines the outer limit of the region of interest. The inner limit is identified by a closed and smoothed polygon connecting several points identified by the operator inside of the vessel lumen near the blood–plaque interface.

5.4.2.3. Edge detection and coordinate transformation

Two edge subimages are generated from the region of interest utilizing Sobel-like edge operators. For computational convenience, the edge subimages are resampled in directions perpendicular to the outlining ellipse. This has the effect of "straightening" the outside boundaries of the regions of interest. These straightened edge subimages are used for construction of the *laminae border detection graph* which is searched to identify the external and internal clastic laminae and the *plaque border detection graph* for identifying the lumen borders.

To calculate edge directions, the original image data corresponding to the laminae and plaque edge subimages are resampled using the same coordinate transformations used to resample the two edge images. Prewitt compass edge operator is applied to the two resampled original images to detect local edge directions.

5.4.2.4. Identification of vessel wall and plaque borders

Graph searching approach to border detection is well understood.[5,105] The key to identifying accurate borders using graph searching is to define an appropriate cost function for nodes in the graph. Since the properties of border pixels forming the external elastic lamina, internal elastic lamina, and plaque differ, separate cost functions were developed for the detection of each border. In contrast to the usual application of graph searching to border detection where cost is inversely related to edge strength, the cost functions in this ultrasound border detection method are related to a specific expected edge pattern and incorporate *a priori* knowledge about cross-sectional arterial anatomy.

5.4.2.5. Identification of the external elastic lamina

Two types of *a priori* information are used to calculate the cost function for the external elastic lamina. The operator-entered outer boundary of the region of interest is used as a rough model for the shape of the external lamina. This is accomplished by identifying the external lamina from the edge subimage after applying the coordinate transformation and by appropriate calculation of node and path costs. Border shapes that mimic the shape of the model are preferred. This is appropriate since the external elastic lamina is known to have an approximately elliptic shape. Because the vessel border is not exactly elliptic and/or the operator-entered ellipse may be inaccurate, the contribution of the model to the cost function represents a compromise between the weight given to the edge information contained in the image data and the weight assigned to the *a priori* information obtained from the shape of the model.

The second type of *a priori* information incorporated in the cost function is the expected double-echo pattern arising from the interfaces of the media and the surrounding external and internal elastic laminae. Costs associated with each node are designed to reflect the degree of match between the local edge configuration and the expected double-echo edge pattern. The expected edge configuration is shown in Figures 6a and 6b. E_l is leading edge of the ultrasound echo response and represents the location of the external elastic lamina. E_t represents the trailing edge of the echo response to the external lamina. I_l and I_t represent the leading and trailing edges of the echo response depicting the internal elastic lamina. In the presence of intimal thickening and plaque development, the echo response from plaque may merge with the internal lamina echo response. In that case, the leading edge I_l may not be detectable in the image. Considering anatomical knowledge about media thickness and the fact that the edge I_l cannot be assumed to be present, the combination of three strong edges I_t, E_l, and E_t located approximately 0.1 mm apart (2–6 pixels in our case) and having appropriate edge directions is given the highest likelihood of indicating the position of the external elastic lamina. As such, the identification of the external elastic lamina is based on searching for edge triplets which form a contiguous circumferential pattern in

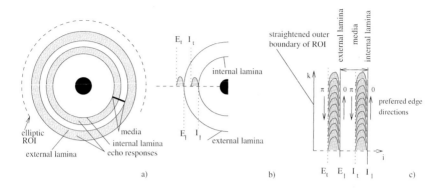

Figure 6. Knowledge-based system for coronary wall and plaque border detection of the University of Iowa. External elastic lamina detection. (left) Ultrasound responses from internal and external elastic laminae form a double-echo pattern. (middle) Idealized echo responses along a radial profile. (right) Leading and trailing edges of echo responses from internal and external elastic laminae in the resampled image.

the original ultrasound image. The position of the external lamina is defined as the location of the echo leading edge E_l (Figure 6c).

More formally, let $f(k, i)$ denote the edge strength of the i-th node on the k-th graph profile of the resampled edge subimage for laminae detection (Figure 6c). Let $d(k, i)$ be its edge direction. The cost $c_E(k, i)$ assigned to a node on a path corresponding to the external lamina depends on the edge triplet or pattern cost $\hat{c}_E(k, i)$ and the direction by which the node is reached. The edge pattern cost is inversely related to edge pattern strength $P(k, i)$:

$$\hat{c}_E(k, i) = \max_{x \in X, y \in Y} \{P(x, y)\} - P(k, i) \tag{1}$$

X, Y are sets of integers ranging from 1 to the width of the region of interest and from 1 to the length of the outer boundary of the region of interest, respectively. They define the size of the rectangular two-dimensional laminae border detection graph. The edge pattern strength $P(k, i)$ is related to the sum of the edge strengths associated with the leading and trailing edges of the echo responses to the external lamina and the trailing edge of the internal lamina response:

$$P(k, i) = E_l(k, i) + E_t(k, i) + I_t(k, i) \tag{2}$$

with

$$E_l(k, i) = \begin{cases} f(k, i) & \text{for } d(k, i) \in [-\pi/2, \pi/2] \\ f(k, i) - dp & \text{otherwise} \end{cases} \tag{3}$$

$$E_t(k, i) = \max_{j=-4,-2} \{f_{Et}(k, i + j)\} \tag{4}$$

$$I_t(k, i) = \max_{j=3,6} \{f_{It}(k, i + j)\} \tag{5}$$

and

$$f_{Et}(k, i) = \begin{cases} f(k, i) & \text{for } d(k, i) \in [\pi/2, 3\pi/2] \\ f(k, i) - dp & \text{otherwise} \end{cases} \tag{6}$$

$$f_{It}(k, i) = \begin{cases} f(k, i) & \text{for } d(k, i) \in [\pi/2, 3\pi/2] \\ f(k, i) - dp & \text{otherwise} \end{cases} \tag{7}$$

The preferred edge directions for leading and trailing edge echo responses are 0 and π respectively (Figure 6c); dp is the penalty used to distinguish between edges with 'appropriate' and 'inappropriate' edge directions. In essence, the edge pattern strength associated with a possible location (k, i) of the external lamina depends on the local edge strength together with nearby edge strengths that potentially correspond with the trailing edges of the echo responses to the internal and external laminae.

The elliptic model for the shape of the external elastic lamina is incorporated in the cost function by modifying node costs when paths are formed. The model corresponds to a straight line in the laminae border detection graph. Therefore, paths in the graph that are not straight represent deviations from the model and are discriminated against by adding a model penalty mp to the node cost. Paths to a node are grouped in two classes according to the direction by which the node is reached from its predecessor. The modified node cost $c_E(k, i)$ is given by

$$c_E(k, i) = \begin{cases} \hat{c}_E(k, i) & \text{if the predecessor's coordinates are } (k - 1, i) \\ \hat{c}_E(k, i) + mp & \text{otherwise} \end{cases} \tag{8}$$

The value of the model penalty mp determines the model's strength. Similar to other model-based border detection strategies, an excessively strong model would force the border to follow the model even when the image data were inconsistent with the model. The appropriate model strength for intravascular ultrasound border detection is determined empirically.

After assigning an appropriate cost $c_E(k, i)$ to each graph node, the optimal path forming a closed boundary in the original image space is searched for in the two-dimensional graph. The optimal path is defined as the path with the minimum sum of costs of all nodes on the path.

5.4.2.6. Identification of the internal elastic lamina

Using the same laminae border detection graph but a different cost function, a search is conducted for the internal lamina border inside of and in proximity to the external lamina border. The cost assigned to a node depends upon its edge strength, its edge direction, and its position with respect to the external lamina border. Information about media thickness is used as *a priori* knowledge. When searching for the internal lamina border, the previously detected external lamina border is used as a model. The model in this case forms a narrow region of support in which the internal border is most likely to be located. The region of support is defined as a 0.2 mm wide strip located 3 to 10 pixels (0.1–0.3 mm) inside the external lamina border. The cost of graph nodes outside the region of support is increased by penalty sp.

The cost $c_I(k, i)$ assigned to a node at position (k, i) is given by:

$$c_I(k, i) = \begin{cases} \hat{c}_I(k, i) & \text{if } 4 \leq (i - j) \leq 11 \\ \hat{c}_I(k, i) + sp & \text{otherwise} \end{cases} \tag{9}$$

where (k, j) are coordinates of the detected external lamina border and

$$\hat{c}_I(k, i) = \max_{x \in X, y \in Y} \{f_{II}(x, y)\} - f_{II}(k, i) \tag{10}$$

with

$$f_{II}(k, i) = \begin{cases} f(k, i) & \text{for } d(k, i) \in [-\pi/2, \pi/2] \\ f(k, i) - dp & \text{otherwise} \end{cases} \tag{11}$$

The preferred edge direction is 0 (Figure 6c) and dp is the directional penalty. The internal elastic lamina border is defined as the minimum cost path through the laminae border detection graph with costs $c_I(k, i)$.

5.4.2.7. Identification of the plaque border

Detection of the plaque border is less difficult than detecting lamina borders since the blood-plaque interface represents the border with the highest contrast in the intravascular ultrasound image. The plaque border is identified using the plaque border detection graph with node costs $c_P(k, i)$ calculated from edge strength and local edge direction:

$$c_P(k, i) = \max_{x \in X', y \in Y'} \{f_{Pl}(x, y)\} - f_{Pl}(k, i) \tag{12}$$

with

$$f_{Pl}(k, i) = \begin{cases} f(k, i) & \text{for } d(k, i) \in [-\pi/2, \pi/2] \\ f(k, i) - dp & \text{otherwise} \end{cases} \tag{13}$$

$f(k, i)$ is the edge strength in the resampled edge subimage for plaque border detection. X', Y' represent the dimensions of the plaque border detection graph, dp is the directional penalty, and the preferred edge direction is 0. The plaque border is defined as the minimum cost path through the plaque border detection graph with costs $c_P(k, i)$.

5.4.2.8. Quantitative evaluation of arterial morphology

External and internal elastic laminae and plaque borders are smoothed using a moving average of 31 border points and mapped back into the original image space as shown in Figure 7. Lumen area, total arterial area (area encompassed by the internal lamina), plaque area, percent area stenosis (fraction of total arterial area occupied by plaque), segmental media thickness, and segmental plaque thickness are then calculated.

In designing our intravascular ultrasound border detection method, we have attempted to mimic the strategies employed by experienced ultrasonographers when attempting to visually identify arterial borders. When the local distribution of image intensities do not allow unambiguous border identification, expert observers will rely upon the *a priori* knowledge they have accumulated about intravascular ultrasound image characteristics. Their final decision about border locations will represent a balance between the clues provided by local image patterns and their expectations about overall image characteristics. It is of course possible that the two will at times conflict and it is thus necessary to make a trade-off between local border detection accuracy and overall analysis reliability. We have made the same sort of trade-off in designing the overall scheme and cost functions used in our border detection method. The resulting method successfully identifies wall and plaque borders in images of fresh cadaveric vessels with a wide variety of atherosclerotic plaques. The computational complexity of the method is modest; processing of an image requires about 7 seconds using an HP 715/100 workstation.

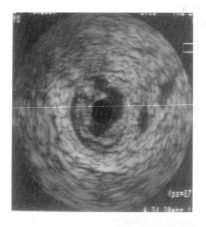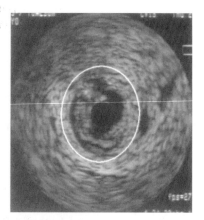

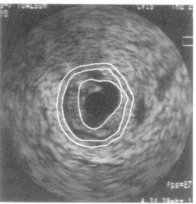

Figure 7. Coronary wall and plaque border detection in single-frame images (the University of Iowa knowledge-based method). (top-left) Original IVUS image. (top-right) Elliptic outline of the region of interest. (bottom) From the outside in: computer-determined external elastic lamina, internal elastic lamina, and lumen borders.

5.4.3. Benefits of Three-dimensional Analysis

The three-dimensional geometry of a stenotic lumen may be visualized during an intravascular ultrasound catheter "pullback" which produces a closely-spaced sequence of high resolution tomographic images.[26] Fractured eccentric plaque, irregular and fissured plaque surfaces, and stretching or thinning of the wall are frequently seen during intravascular ultrasound imaging but are often missed in angiography.[65,91,106,107]

An important limitation of serial studies with intravascular ultrasound which compare initial findings with a follow-up result[108–110] is the fact that the sites of ultrasound measurement are not always identical. This can be explained by the lack of the third dimension in conventional two-dimensional intravascular ultrasound images.[111] Three-dimensional reconstruction of intravascular ultrasound images allows a much more reliable serial evaluation at identical sites of the coronary artery and the measurement of plaque volume. On-line analysis of the target lesion and the reference segment may facilitate and guide coronary interventions, giving essential information concerning the optimal type and size of interventional devices.[112] The longitudinal reconstruction of coronary arteries provides additional insight into plaque geometry and facilitates the analysis of dissections.[113–114] An excellent correlation with histology has been described by Coy *et al.* in the evaluation of length and depth of dissections.[115] After stent implantation the intra-stent dimensions can be evaluated by three-dimensional intravascular ultrasound,[50] facilitating the detection of incomplete stent apposition. The value and specific usefulness of three-dimensional on-line reconstruction in planning and guiding coronary stenting has recently been reported.[116] In directional coronary atherectomy the orientation of the cutter in relation to side-branches and the detection of deep or spiral cuts may be facilitated by three-dimensionally reconstructed ultrasound.[117] A reliable serial evaluation of progression/regression of atherosclerosis depends critically on the correct matching of the images. Three-dimensional reconstruction facilitates the process of matching and increases the accuracy of comparisons. Volumetric measurement of lumen and plaque[85,118–122] may be an alternative to the measurement of minimal luminal area, since plaque volume reflects changes in total plaque burden and appears to show a higher reproducibility than area measurements.[118] Although the hemodynamic significance of a coronary plaque is most closely correlated to the minimal cross-sectional area,[123] it is likely that plaque volume may better reflect the process of progression or regression of atherosclerosis than area measurements, performed at the site of the minimal luminal area. The applicability of volumetric plaque analysis in directional coronary atherectomy has recently been proven by Dhawale *et al.*[120]

5.4.4. Approaches to Three-dimensional Analysis of IVUS Image Data

Several sequential processing steps have to be performed in order to obtain a reliable three-dimensional reconstruction of the conventional two-dimensional intravascular ultrasound images. The gain settings must always be optimized before the basic ultrasound images are acquired since most of the reconstruction programs allow the display of the full range of gray scale information (volume rendered display). Side-branches or spots of calcium are always used as topographic landmarks. Starting distal of the stenosis, the ultrasound catheter is pulled back through the coronary artery segment which is subject to reconstruction. Several pull-back methods have been described and applied.[118,124] Presently, the continuous pull-back at a uniform-speed, resulting in an equidistant spacing of adjacent images,[125] is the most common approach. A modified concept is the ECG-gated video labeling, which marks certain video frames during a uniform pull-back, triggered by the R-wave of the ECG.[126] Alternatively, a stepping motor gated by an ECG-signal can be used for a non-uniform stepwise withdrawal of the ultrasound imaging catheter. Using a dynamic three-dimensional reconstruction system, initially designed for the reconstruction of transthoracic or transesophageal echocardiography (TomTec GmbH, Munich, Germany),[127–129] the moving coronary artery can be dynamically visualized during the cardiac cycle.[130] Segmentation is at present mainly achieved by the application of voxel-based algorithms, discriminating between the blood-pool inside the lumen and structures of the vessel wall.[131–133] The threshold method, providing a segmentation based on the definition of thresholds for lumen and vessel wall in the scale of gray levels, has been used to obtain the first reliable three-dimensional reconstructions of intravascular ultrasound images.[94,114] Another approach is an algorithm for statistical pattern recognition (EchoQuantTM, Indec, Capitola, CA, USA).[133,134] This algorithm is able to distinguish between the patterns of the flowing blood inside the lumen and the vessel wall and may be used to remove the pixels of the blood pool. Application of the algorithm may sometimes be hampered by the quality of the basic images,[134,135] however, the automated detection can be checked and manually corrected.

The knowledge-based contour detection system described detects the plaque borders and the internal and external elastic laminae. The efforts to develop a fully automated three-dimensional intravascular ultrasound border detection method now focus on utilizing the contextual information from subsequent image frames both in temporal and spatial image sequences. A preliminary implementation of a fully automated method for coronary wall and plaque border detection in short pressure sequences and catheter pullbacks suggested feasibility of such an approach both *in vitro* and *in vivo*.[136,137]

The set of three-dimensional image data can be shown in different display formats. A sagittal (longitudinal) format, a lumen cast display and a cylindrical view — a coronary segment opened longitudinally with both halves tilted back giving an open "clam-shell" view — are the most significant display formats.[126] The quantification features of the different three-dimensional reconstruction programs differ considerably. To date only the contour-detection approach permits the measurement of plaque volume *in vivo* in clinical intravascular ultrasound studies.[118]

5.4.5. Contour Detection Approach to Three-dimensional IVUS Image Analysis

A contour detection method developed at the Thoraxcenter and Erasmus University Rotterdam is specifically directed at the analysis of three-dimensional IVUS image sequences obtained from motorized pullbacks of the ultrasound catheter. Volumetric measurements can be based on regional analysis of arterial lumen and plaque in each ultrasonic cross-sectional image.

The method is based on the application of a minimum cost algorithm[138] that permits the identification of the boundaries between the lumen and plaque as well as the plaque-media complex and adventitia.[84,85,118,133,139] The luminal borders are defined by the leading edge of the intima or plaque echo response. To measure the size of the total cross-sectional area of the artery, the ultrasound interface between media and adventitia is determined. The plaque area is calculated by subtracting the lumen area from the total arterial area. Plaque or lumen volumes V are calculated as a sum of products of slice thickness H and plaque area A_i in N individual IVUS frames of the pullback sequence.

$$V = \sum_{i=1}^{N} A_i H \qquad (14)$$

Using a frame grabber with the maximum digitization rate of 20 frames/s, the length of the reconstructed segment is defined by the speed of the motorized pullback. The pixel size depending on the magnification of the ultrasound system ranges from 0.026 to 0.036 mm. The contour detection method consists of three major steps.[84] First, the IVUS image sequence is modeled in a volumetric space[132] and two perpendicular cut planes which are parallel to the longitudinal axis of the vessel segment are interactively selected and two longitudinal images are reconstructed (Figure 8). Second, the dynamic programming based minimum cost algorithm is used to detect lumen contour and media contour in the longitudinal images. This processing step is first performed automatically and then points can be manually added to force the contour to pass through them (interactive correction). Dynamic programming techniques are used to determine the new optimal longitudinal contours after each manual interaction what permits frequent updates of the display. As a result of the longitudinal border detection, four individual edge points are derived for each contour in each IVUS frame and are

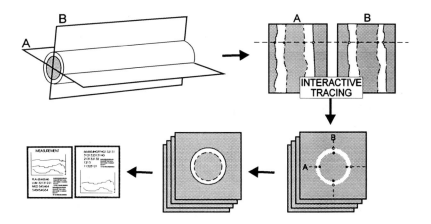

Figure 8. Contour detection system of the Thoraxcenter Rotterdam. Two perpendicular longitudinal images (A, B) defined by perpendicular cut planes in the volumetric space. Based on the application of a minimum cost algorithm the longitudinal contours are interactively traced in the longitudinal images. Four edge points for each contour are derived from the longitudinal contours and used as fixed constraints, guiding the final contour detection in the individual cross-sectional ultrasound images. As the last step, the cross-sectional contours can be checked and manual correction may be performed.

used as fixed constraints guiding the third step of the contour detection process, in which lumen and media contours are automatically detected in individual cross-sectional ultrasound images using a minimum cost dynamic programming search in the straightened graph. Inverted edge strength is used to define nodal costs outside the four nodes representing hard constraints, the four constraining points are represented by very low cost nodes in the graph. Finally, the optimal borders identified in individual frames are interpolated and form continuous lumen and media surfaces. The entire process is demonstrated in Figure 8.

5.5. PERFORMANCE OF INTRAVASCULAR IMAGE ANALYSIS METHODS

5.5.1. Performance of the Knowledge-based Method for Coronary Wall and Plaque Border Detection

To evaluate accuracy of the coronary wall and plaque border detection algorithm described in Section 5.4.2,[140,141] the method was applied to

38 intravascular ultrasound images acquired from 24 fresh cadaveric hearts in which post-mortem angiography showed no discrete stenoses in the proximal left anterior descending coronary artery. Under fluoroscopic guidance, a 4.3 French (1.43 mm) intracoronary ultrasound 30 MHz imaging catheter (CVIS, Sunnyvale, CA) was introduced into the cannulated coronary ostium over an angioplasty guidewire. The catheter was moved down the coronary artery to identify an eccentric plaque which is typically seen just after the bifurcation of the left circumflex coronary artery. The IVUS images recorded using S-VHS videotape were digitized at an image resolution of 0.03 mm/pixel.

To assess the performance of our border detection method, we compared automatically detected laminae and plaque borders with carefully determined manually-identified borders which were used as an independent standard. To objectively evaluate the accuracy of our border detection method, we compared lumen area, plaque area, and segmental plaque thickness obtained from computer-detected borders to measures obtained from observer-defined borders. We also directly compared computer-detected and observer-defined borders by calculating maximum and root-mean-square (rms) border positioning errors.

All 38 intravascular ultrasound images were successfully analyzed by the border detection method. Computer-identified lumen areas correlated very well with observer-defined lumen areas ($r = 0.96$, $y = 1.02x + 0.52$, Figure 9a). Computer-identified plaque areas also correlated very well with observer-defined plaque areas ($r = 0.95$, $y = 1.07x - 0.48$, Figure 9b). The average absolute (unsigned) error of plaque thickness measurement was 0.16 ± 0.04 mm, the average signed error of plaque thickness was 0.00 ± 0.10 mm. Average maximum and rms border positioning errors for the external and internal laminae and plaque borders were 0.32 ± 0.09 mm and 0.08 ± 0.02 mm, respectively. To appreciate the small size of these border position errors, one needs to remember that the maximal obtainable accuracy is of the order of one wavelength of the transmitted ultrasound.[142] At a wavelength of 30 MHz, the theoretical limiting accuracy is 0.05 mm. Thus, the laminae and plaque border detection were highly accurate.

Figures 10 and 11 show examples of two intravascular ultrasound images, computer-detected internal and external elastic laminae and plaque borders, and the borders defined by expert observers. The computer-defined borders closely approximate the borders defined by the expert observer.

5.5.2. Performance of the Contour Detection Method for Three-dimensional IVUS Analysis

To assess the accuracy of the contour detection method, it was applied to IVUS images of a tubular phantom of known dimensions. A tubular paraffin

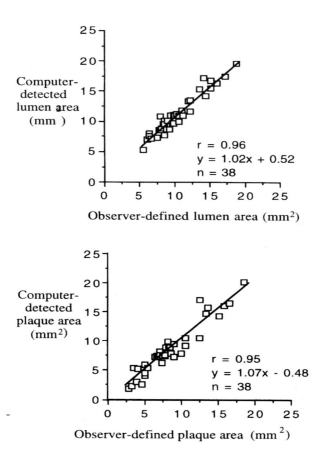

Figure 9. Comparison of computer-detected (the University of Iowa knowledge-based method) and observer-defined lumen area (above) and plaque area (below).

phantom with a circular lumen and a stepwise increase in diameter (2, 3, 4, and 5 mm diameters formed four 5 mm long segments) was fixed inside an acrylate tube. The phantom dimensions were optically calibrated using a calibrated stereo microscope. Five pullbacks were performed in the tubular phantom *in vitro* and recorded on a S-VHS video tape. Ultrasound measurements of the phantom lumen volume showed a high correlation with the true volumes of the four phantom segments ($r = 0.99$, $y = 1.02x - 0.42$, $SEE = 11.7 \, \text{mm}^3$, $n = 20$), with mean signed differences between $-0.04 \, \text{mm}^3$ and $-1.69 \, \text{mm}^3$ for the four phantom segments of constant diameter.

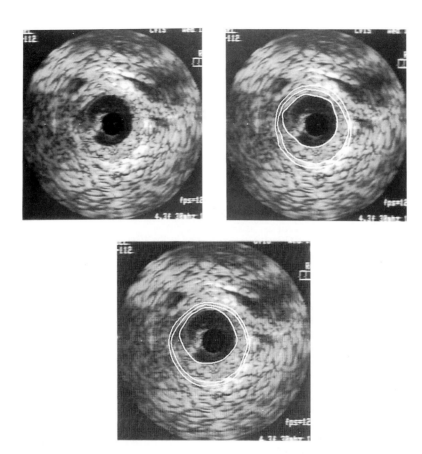

Figure 10. Intravascular ultrasound border detection in a diseased coronary vessel using the knowledge-based method. (top-left) Original image showing plaque thickening at the 2- to 9-o'clock position. (top-right) Computer-determined internal and external elastic laminae and plaque borders. (bottom) Manually-identified internal and external elastic laminae and plaque borders.

Intra- and inter-observer variability of plaque and lumen volume measurements *in vivo* were determined in 20 atherosclerotic coronary arteries. The IVUS images were obtained during uniform (1 mm/s) motorized pullbacks of 2.9F 30 MHz mechanical catheters (Microview, CVIS, Sunnyvale, CA). This type of IVUS catheters has a distal echo-transparent common lumen to accommodate either the guidewire or the IVUS transducer but never both at the same time. Using 20 IVUS examinations of human

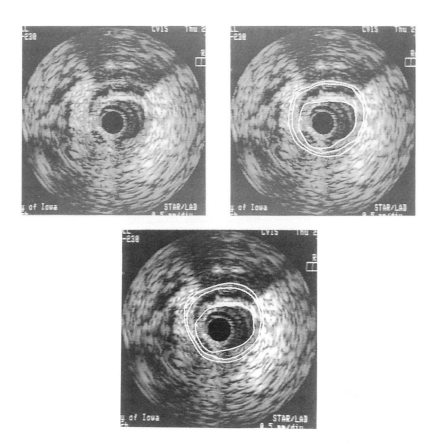

Figure 11. Intravascular ultrasound border detection in a diseased coronary vessel using the knowledge-based method. (top-left) Original image showing plaque thickening at the 9- to 7-o'clock position. (top-right) Computer-determined internal and external elastic laminae and plaque borders. (bottom) Manually-identified internal and external elastic laminae and plaque borders.

coronary arteries *in vivo* (each: 200 images/20 mm segments), intra- and inter-observer variability of the quantification method were studied. The IVUS pullback sequences imaged 20 mm long coronary segments and were acquired before, directly after, or at follow up after various catheter-based interventions reflecting the current routine clinical application of IVUS imaging at the Thoraxcenter. A clinical example *in vivo* is shown in Figure 12. The IVUS examinations were recorded on a video tape and analyzed off line. The ability to display the cross-sectional plus two

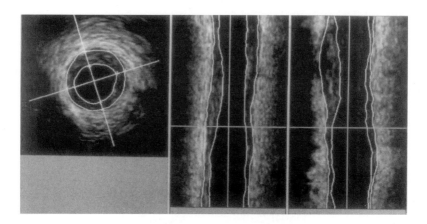

Figure 12. Clinical *in vivo* examination using the quantitative analysis system of the Thoraxcenter Rotterdam. The position of an individual cross-sectional IVUS image in the longitudinal sections is indicated by a horizontal cursor line that can be used to scroll through the entire series of cross-sectional images.

longitudinal views simultaneously facilitated the contour detection process. Volumetric segmentation of IVUS pullbacks may serve for three-dimensional visualization of coronary segments. Although three-dimensional rendering is not necessary for reliable quantification, it offers a completely new visualization of coronary disease morphology *in vivo* (Figure 13). The intra- and inter-observer measurements *in vivo* showed high correlation with $r = 0.99$ for lumen and plaque volumes (Figure 14). The inter-observer mean signed differences of lumen and plaque volume measurements were low: -0.89 ± 4.95 mm^3 and 1.51 ± 4.86 mm^3, respectively.

The findings demonstrate that the contour detection based IVUS analysis system performs an accurate volumetric quantification and can be used to perform highly reproducible measurements of plaque and lumen volume in three-dimensionally reconstructed IVUS images *in vivo*.[118] Additionally, the reproducibility of area measurements is high as demonstrated in the 4000 IVUS image frames.[118] The percent standard deviations of the signed inter-observer differences were relatively lower for volumetric measurements. This suggests that the volumetric approach reduces the variability of area measurements by partially averaging out overestimation and underestimation of area measurements in individual cross-sectional IVUS images.

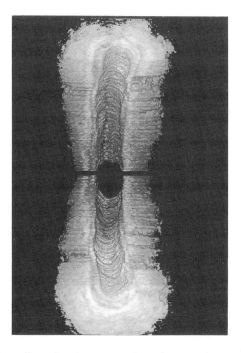

Figure 13. Three-dimensional reconstruction of a coronary segment *in vivo* after balloon angioplasty processed with the contour detection system of the Thoraxcenter Rotterdam. The pixels of the blood pool have been removed and a surface-rendered cylindrical view is presented. However, the three-dimensional rendering is not necessary for reliable quantification.

5.6. CONCLUSION

Intravascular ultrasound is a promising new imaging method for evaluating coronary artery anatomy. Because of its ability to directly image coronary lumen and wall cross-sectional dimensions and to assess the composition of atherosclerotic plaque, intravascular ultrasound may ultimately replace angiography as the gold standard in evaluating coronary artery disease.[26,28] Although there is substantial and growing interest in quantitative analysis of intravascular ultrasound images, only very limited progress has been reported in the literature on the development of fully automated methods for identifying wall and lumen/plaque borders. We described methodology and validation of two distinct computerized approaches to IVUS image analysis developed at two leading research centers, at the University of Iowa in Iowa City, USA and the Thoraxcenter of the Erasmus University Rotterdam,

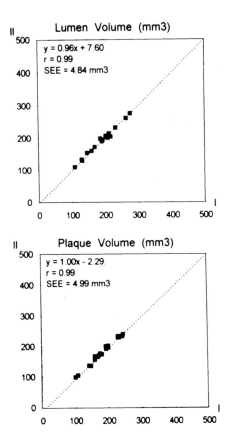

Figure 14. Inter-observer variability of volumetric measurements *in vivo* (the Thoraxcenter method). The results of linear regression analysis comparing lumen and plaque volume measurements of two independent analysts (I and II) are presented. The dotted lines mark the lines of identity.

The Netherlands. Computer-detected borders showed very good agreement with phantoms and manually-traced borders as well as a high reproducibility of cross-sectional and volumetric measurements. Nevertheless, some limitations of two-dimensional and three-dimensionally analyzed intravascular ultrasound images still remain,[111,143] such as the compression of the plaque by the ultrasound catheter at the site of vessel curvature. Artifacts resulting from the movement of the ultrasound catheter during the cardiac cycle and systolic-diastolic changes in vessel dimensions can be minimized by the use of an ECG-gated pull-back system.[111,117] Combined use of biplane angiography and ultrasound data, provided by the contour detection method may help to display the real vessel geometry and correct for the image distortion,[144] caused by vessel curvature and catheter bends,[145] in the not too distant future.

Intravascular ultrasound offers a unique *in vivo* visualization of coronary artery morphology with direct clinical utility. Ultrasound-guided coronary interventions can be performed safely with excellent results. Intravascular ultrasound image quality is now rapidly improving due to the introduction of new catheters and ultrasound signal processing techniques. These advances should facilitate the development of fully automated analysis procedures. Assuming continued technical progress, similar to that of the previous years, computer analysis of intravascular ultrasound images will likely become a significant research and clinical tool in the hands of the coming generation of interventional cardiologists.

5.7. ACKNOWLEDGMENTS

This work was supported in part by the National American Heart Association, American Heart Association — Iowa Affiliate, Carver Scientific Research Initiative Grants Program, Central Investment Fund for Research Enhancement of the University of Iowa. Dr. von Birgelen is the recipient of a research fellowship of the German Research Society (DFG).

5.8. REFERENCES

1. Collins, S.M. and D.J. Skorton, editors, 1986, *Cardiac Imaging and Image Processing.* McGraw Hill, New York.
2. Marcus, M.L., H.R. Schelbert, D.J. Skorton and G.L. Wolf, 1991, *Cardiac Imaging.* W.B. Saunders, Philadelphia.
3. Liebson, P.R. and L.W. Klein, 1991, Intravascular ultrasound in coronary atherosclerosis: A new approach to clinical assessment. *Am. Heart J.*, **123**, 1643–1660.
4. de Feyter, P.J., C. Di Mario and P.W. Serruys, 1995, *Quantitative Coronary Imaging.* Barjesteh, Meeuwes & Co., Rotterdam.
5. Sonka, M. and S.M. Collins, ????, Automated analysis of coronary angiograms. In C.T. Leondes, editor, *Medical Imaging Techniques and Applications.* Gordon and Breach. In this Gordon and Breach series.
6. Marcus, M.L., D.J. Skorton, M.R. Johnson, S.M. Collins, D.G. Harrison and R.E. Kerber, 1988, Visual estimates of percent diamater coronary stenosis: A battered gold standard. *J. Am. Coll. Cardiol.*, **11**, 882–885.
7. Mancini, G.B.J., 1991, Applications of digital angiography to the coronary circulation. In M.L. Marcus and D.J. Skorton, editors, *Cardiac Imaging: Principles and Practice*, pp. 310–347. W.B. Saunders, Philadelphia.
8. Reiber, J.H.C., P.W. Serruys and J.D. Barth, 1991, Quantitative coronary angiography. In M.L. Marcus, H.R. Schelbert, D.J. Skorton and G.L. Wolf, editors, *Cardiac Imaging*, pp. 211–280. W.B. Saunders, Philadelphia.

9. Nissen, S.E., J.C. Gurley, C.L. Grines, D.C. Booth, R. McClure, M. Berk, C. Ficher and A.N. DeMaria, 1991, Intravascular ultrasound assessment of lumen size and wall morphology in normal subjects and patients with coronary artery disease. *Circulation*, **84**, 1087–1099.

10. Hausmann, D., A.J.S. Lundkvist, G.J. Friedrich, W.L. Mullen, P.J. Fitzgerald and P.G. Yock, 1994, Intracoronary ultrasound imaging: Intraobserver and interobserver variability of morphometric measurements. *Am. Heart J.*, **128**, 674–680.

11. Escaned, J., J. Haase, D.P. Foley, C. Di Mario, A. Den Boer, E.M. van Swijndregt and P.W. Serruys, 1994, Videodensitometry in percutaneous coronary interventions: A critical appraisal of its contributions and limitations. In *Quantitative coronary angiography in clinical practice*, pp. 69–87, Dordrecht-Boston-London. Kluwer Academic Publishers.

12. Keane, D. and P.W. Serruys, 1995, Quantitative coronary angiography: An integral component of interventional cardiology. In *Current review of interventional cardiology, 2nd edition*, in press, Philadelphia USA. Current Medicine.

13. Mancini, G.B.J., 1991, Quantitative coronary arteriographic methods in the interventional catheterization laboratory: An update and perspective. *J. Am. Coll. Cardiol.*, **17**(6), 23B–33B.

14. Davidson, C.J., W.L. Mullen, B.A. Bergelson, R.F. Fishman, M.A. Parker, A. Schaechter, S.N. Meyers and C.L. Tommaso, 1994, For the GUIDE-II-Investigators (abst). *J. Am. Coll. Cardiol.*, **23**, 174A.

15. Bom, N., W. Li, A.F.W. van der Steen, C.L. de Korte, E.J. Gussenhoven, C. von Birgelen, C.T. Lancee and J.R.T.C. Roelandt, 1995, Intravascular ultrasound: Technical update 1995. In P.J. de Feyter, C. Di Mario and P.W. Serruys, editors, *Quantitative Coronary Imaging*, pp. 89–106. Barjesteh, Meeuwes & Co., Rotterdam.

16. Siebes, M., R.R. Chada, X. Zhang, M. Sonka, C.R. McKay and S.M. Collins, 1994, Biomechanical characterization of blood vessel and plaque from intravascular ultrasound images. In *Physiology and Function from Multidimensional Images, Proceedings SPIE Vol. 2168*, pp. 33–42, Bellingham, WA, SPIE.

17. Sonka, M., X. Zhang, M. Siebes, R.R. Chada, C.R. McKay and S.M. Collins, 1994, Automated detection of wall and plaque borders in intravascular ultrasound images. In *Physiology and Function from Multidimensional Images, Proceedings SPIE Vol. 2168*, pp. 13–22, Bellingham, WA, SPIE.

18. Hodgson, J.M., S.D. Graham, A.D. Savakus, S.G. Dame, D.N. Stephens, P.S. Dhillon, D. Brands, H. Sheehan and M.J. Eberle, 1989, Clinical percutaneous imaging of coronary anatomy using an over-the-wire ultrasound catheter system. *Int. J. Card. Imag.*, **4**, 187–193.

19. Mallery, J.A., J.M. Tobis, J. Griffith, J. Gessert, M. McRae, O. Moussabeck, M. Bessen, M. Moriuchi and W.L. Henry, 1990, Assessment of normal and atherosclerotic arterial wall thickness with an intravascular ultrasound catheter. *Am. Heart J.*, **119**, 1392–1400.

20. Davidson, C.J., Davidson, K.H. Sheikh, J.K. Harrison, S.I. Himmelstein, M.E. Leithe, K.B. Kisslo and T.M. Bashore, 1990, Intravascular ultrasonography versus digital subtraction angiography: A human *in vivo* comparison of vessel size and morphology. *J. Am. Coll. Cardiol.*, **16**, 633–636.

21. Hodgson, J.M., S.P. Graham, H. Sheenan and A.D. Savakus, 1990, Percutaneous intracoronary ultrasound imaging: Initial applications in patients. *Echocardiography*, **7**, 403–413.

22. Potkin, B.N., A.L. Bartorelli, J.M. Gessert, R.F. Neville, Y. Almagor, W.C. Robberts and M.B. Leon, 1990, Coronary artery imaging with intravascular high-frequency ultrasound. *Circulation*, **81**, 1575–1585.

23. Fitzgerald, P.J., F.G.St. Goar, A.J. Connolly, F.J. Pinto, M.E. Billingham, R.L. Popp and P.G. Yock, 1992, Intravascular ultrasound imaging of coronary arteries. Is three layers the norm? *Circulation*, **86**, 154–158.

24. McKay, C.R., B.F. Waller, I. Gessert, M. Catellier, S.R. Fleagle and M.L. Marcus, 1989, Quantitative analysis of coronary artery morphology using intracoronary high frequency ultrasound: Validation by histology and quantitative coronary angiography (abstract). *J. Am. Coll. Cardiol.*, **13**, 228A.

25. Gussenhoven, E.J., C.E. Essed, C.T. Lancee, F. Mastik, P. Frietman, F.C. van Egmond, J. Reiber, H. Bosch, H. van Urk, J. Roelandt and N. Bom, 1989, Arterial wall characteristics determined by intravascular ultrasound imaging: An *in vitro* study. *J. Am. Coll. Cardiol.*, **14**, 947–952.

26. Tobis, J.M., 1991, Intravascular ultrasound: A fantastic voyage. *Circulation*, **84**, 2190–2192.

27. Pandian, N.G., A. Kreis and A. Weintraub, 1990, Real-time intravascular imaging in humans. *Am. J. Cardiol.*, **65**, 1392–1396.

28. Waller, B.F., C.A. Pinkerton and J.D. Slack, 1992, Intravascular ultrasound: A histological study of vessels during life. The new 'gold standard' for vascular imaging. *Circulation*, **85**, 2305–2309.

29. Yock, P.G., P.J. Fitzgerald and D.T. Linker, 1991, Intravascular ultrasound guidance for catheter-based coronary interventions. *J. Am. Coll. Cardiol.*, **17**, 39B–45B.

30. Gerber, T.C., R. Erbel, G. Goerge, J. Ge, H.J. Rupprecht and J. Meyer, 1994, Extent of atherosclerosis and remodeling of the left main coronary artery determined by intravascular ultrasound. *Am. J. Cardiol.*, **73**, 666–671.

31. Hodgson, J.M., K.G. Reddy, R. Suneja, R.N. Nair, E.J. Lesnefsky and H.M. Sheehan, 1993, Intracoronary ultrasound imaging: Correlation of plaque morphology with angiography, clinical syndrome and procedural results in patients undergoing coronary angioplasty. *J. Am. Coll. Cardiol.*, **21**, 35–44.

32. Goar, F.G.St., F.J. Pinto, E.L. Alderman, H.A. Valantine, J.S. Schroeder, S.Z. Gao, E.B. Stinson and R.L. Popp, 1992, Intracoronary ultrasound in cardiac transplant recipients: *In vivo* evidence of angiographically silent intimal thickening. *Circulation*, **85**, 979–987.

33. Yock, P.G. and D.T. Linker, 1990, Intravascular ultrasound. Looking below the surface of vascular disease. *Circulation*, **81**, 1715–1718.

34. Ge, J., R. Erbel, H.J. Rupprecht, L. Koch, P. Kearney, G. Goerge, M. Haude and J. Meyer, 1994, Comparison of intravascular ultrasound and angiography in the assessment of myocardial bridging. *Circulation*, **89**, 1725–1732.

35. Yamagishi, M., K. Miyatake, J. Tamai, S. Nakatani, J. Kojama and S.E. Nissen, 1994, Intravascular ultrasound detection of atherosclerosis at the site of focal vasospasm in angiographically normal or minimally narrowed coronary segments. *J. Am. Coll. Cardiol.*, **23**, 352–357.

36. Bissing, M.S., S. DeJong, P. Thomas, K. Spencer and C.R. McKay, 1994, Identification of eccentric lesions and lipid laden plaques by IVUS: Validation by quantitative histology in fresh cadaveric hearts (abstract). *Circulation*, **90**, I–551.

37. The GUIDE Trial Investigators, 1994, IVUS-determined predictors of restenosis in PTCA and DCA: An interim report from the guide trial, Phase II (abstract). *Circulation*, **90**, I–23.

38. Glagov, S., E. Weisenberg, C.K. Zaris, R. Stancunavicius and G.J. Kolettis, 1987, Compensatory enlargement of human atherosclerotic coronary arteries. *New Engl. J. Med.*, **316**, 1371–1375.

39. Stiel, G.M., L.S.G. Stiel, J. Schofer, K. Donath and D.G. Mathey, 1989, Impact of compensatory enlargement of atherosclerotic coronary arteries on angiographic assessment of coronary artery disease. *Circulation*, **80**, 1603–1609.

40. McPherson, D.D., L.F. Hiratzka, W.C. Lamberth, B. Brandt, M. Hunt, R.A. Kieso, M.L. Marcus and R.E. Kerber, 1987, Delineation of the extent of coronary atherosclerosis by high-frequency epicardial echocardiography. *New Engl. J. Med.*, **316**, 301–309.

41. Hermiller, J.B., C.E. Buller, A.N. Tenaglia, K.B. Kisslo, H.R. Phillips, T.M. Bashore, R.S. Stack and D.J. Davidson, 1993, Unrecognized left main coronary artery disease in patients undergoing interventional procedures. *Am. J. Cardiol.*, **71**, 173–176.

42. McPherson, D.D., S.J. Sirna, L.F. Hiratzka, L. Thorpe, M.L. Armstrong, M.L. Marcus and R.E. Kerber, 1991, Coronary arterial remodeling studied by high-frequency epicardial echocardiography: An early compensatory mechanism in patients with obstructive coronary atherosclerosis. *J. Am. Coll. Cardiol.*, **17**, 79–86.

43. Ge, J., R. Erbel, J. Zamorano, L. Koch, P. Kearney, G. Goerge, T. Gerber and J. Meyer, 1993, Coronary artery remodeling in atherosclerotic disease: An intravascular ultrasonic study *in vivo*. *Coronary Artery Disease*, **4**, 981–986.

44. Hermiller, J.B., A.N. Tenaglia, K.B. Kisslo, H.R. Phillips, T.M. Bashore, R.S. Stack and C.J. Davidson, 1993, *In vivo* validation of compensatory enlargement of atherosclerotic coronary arteries. *Am. J. Cardiol.*, **71**, 665–668.

45. Losordo, D.W., K. Rosenfield, J. Kaufman, A. Pieczek and J.M. Isner, 1994, Focal compensatory enlargement of human arteries in response to progressive atherosclerosis. *In vivo* documentation using intravascular ultrasound. *Circulation*, **89**, 2570–2577.

46. Gupta, M., A.J. Connolly, B.Q. Zhu, R.E. Sievers, K. Sudhir, Y.P. Sun, W.W. Parmley, P.J. Fitzgerald and P.G. Yock, 1992, Quantitative analysis of progression and regression of atherosclerosis by intravascular ultrasound: Validation in a rabbit model (abstract). *Circulation*, **86**, I–518.

47. Lassetter, J.E., R.C. Krall, D.S. Moddrelle and R.D. Jenkins, 1992, Morphologic changes of the arterial wall during regression of experimental atherosclerosis (abstract). *Circulation*, **86**, I–518.

48. Kimura, B.J., P.J. Fitzgerald, K. Sudhir, T.M. Amidon, B.L. Strunk and P.G. Yock, 1992, Guidance of directional coronary atherectomy by intracoronary ultrasound imaging. *Am. Heart J.*, **124**, 1365–1369.

49. Ellis, S.G., N.B. De Cesare, C.A. Pinkerton, P. Withlow, III S.B. King, Z.B.M. Ghazzal, A.J. Kereiakes, J.J. Popma, K.K. Menke, E.J. Topol and D.R. Holmes, 1991, Relation of stenosis morphology and clinical presentation to the procedural results of directional coronary atherectomy. *Circulation*, **84**, 644–653.

50. Mintz, G.S., B.N. Potkin, G. Keren, L.F. Satler, A.D. Pichard, K.M. Kent, J.J. Popma and M.B. Leon, 1992, Intravascular ultrasound evaluation of the effect of rotational atherectomy in obstructive atherosclerotic coronary artery disease. *Circulation*, **86**, 1383–1393.

51. Honye, J., D.J. Mahon, C.J. White, S.R. Ramee, J.B. Wallis, A. Al-Zarka and J.M. Tobis, 1992, Morphological effects of coronary balloon angioplasty *in vivo* assessed by intravascular ultrasound imaging. *Circulation*, **85**, 1012–1025.

52. Friedrich, G.J., N.Y. Moes, V.A. Muhlberger, C. Gabl, G. Mikuz, D. Hausmann, P.J. Fitzgerald and P.G. Yock, 1994, Detection of intralesional calcium by intracoronary ultrasound depends on the histologic pattern. *Am. Heart J.*, **128**, 435–441.

53. Benkeser, P.J., A.L. Churchwell, C. Lee and D.M. Abouelnasr, 1993, Resolution limitations in intravascular ultrasound imaging. *J. Am. Soc. Echocardiogr.*, **6**, 158–165.

54. Hermans, W.R.M., B.J. Rensing, D.P. Foley, J.W. Deckers, W. Rutsch, H. Emanuelsson, N. Danchin, W. Wijns, F. Chappuis and P.W. Serruys, 1992, Therapeutic dissection after successful coronary angioplasty: No influence on restenosis or on clinical outcome. A study in 693 patients. *J. Am. Coll. Cardiol.*, **20**, 767–780.

55. Leimgruber, P.P., G.S. Roubin, H.V. Anderson, *et al.*, 1985, Influence of intimal dissection on restenosis after successful coronary angioplasty. *Circulation*, **72**, 530–535.

56. Tenaglia, A.N., C.E. Buller, K.B. Kisslo, H.R. Phillips and R.S. Stack, 1992, Intracoronary ultrasound predictors of adverse outcomes after coronary artery interventions. *J. Am. Coll. Cardiol.*, **20**, 1385–1390.

57. Potkin, B.N., G. Keren, G.S. Mintz, P.C. Douek, A.D. Pichard, L.F. Satler, K.M. Kent and M.B. Leon, 1992, Arterial response to balloon coronary angioplasty: An intravascular ultrasound study. *J. Am. Coll. Cardiol.*, **20**, 942–951.

58. Mintz, G.S., A.D. Pichard, J.A. Kovach, K.M. Kent, L.F. Satler, P.J. Saturnino, J.J. Popma and M.B. Leon, 1994, Impact of preintervention intravascular ultrasound imaging on transcatheter treatment strategies in coronary artery disease. *Am. J. Cardiol.*, **73**, 423–430.

59. Kovach, J.A., G.S. Mintz, A.D. Pichard, K.M. Kent, J.J. Popma, L.F. Satler and M.B. Leon, 1993, Sequential intravascular ultrasound characterization of the mechanisms of rotational atherectomy and adjunct balloon angioplasty. *J. Am. Coll. Cardiol.*, **22**, 1024–1032.

60. Mintz, G.S., J.J. Popma, C.J. Ditrano, J. Mackenzie and L.F. Satler, 1993, Intravascular ultrasound vs. quantitative coronary angiography: A statistical comparison of 538 consecutive target lesions (abstract). *Circulation*, **88**, I–411.

61. The, S.H.K., E.J. Gussenhoven, Y. Zhong, W. Li, F. van Egmond, H. Pieterman, H. van Urk, P. Gerritsen, C. Borst, R.A. Wilson and N. Bom, 1992, Effect of balloon angioplasty on femoral artery evaluated with intravascular ultrasound imaging. *Circulation*, **86**, 483–493.

62. Tenaglia, A.N., C.E. Buller, K.B. Kisslo, R.S. Stack and C.J. Davidson, 1992, Mechanisms of balloon angioplasty and directional coronary atherectomy as assessed by intracoronary ultrasound. *J. Am. Coll. Cardiol.*, **20**, 685–691.

63. Losordo, D.W., K. Rosenfield, A. Pieczek, K. Baker, M. Harding and J.M. Isner, 1992, How does angioplasty work? Serial analysis of human iliac arteries using intravascular ultrasound. *Circulation*, **86**, 1845–1858.

64. Braden, G.A., D.M. Herrington, T.R. Downes, M.A. Kutcher and W.C. Little, 1994, Qualitative and quantitative contrasts in the mechanisms of lumen enlargement by coronary balloon angioplasty and directional coronary atherectomy. *J. Am. Coll. Cardiol.*, **23**, 40–48.

65. Gerber, T.C., R. Erbel, G. Goerge, J. Ge, H. Rupprecht and J. Meyer, 1992, Classification of morphologic effects of percutaneous transluminal coronary angioplasty assessed by intravascular ultrasound. *Am. J. Cardiol.*, **70**, 1546–1554.

66. Tobis, J.M., J.A. Mallery, D. Mahon, K. Lehmann, P. Zalesky, J. Griffith, J. Gessert, M. Moriuchi, M. McRae, M.L. Dwyer, N. Greep and W.L. Henry, 1991, Intravascular ultrasound imaging of human arteries *in vivo*. *Circulation*, **83**, 913–926.

67. Garrand, T.J., G.S. Mintz, J.J. Popma, S.A. Lewis, A.N. Vaughn and M.B. Leon, 1993, Intravascular ultrasound diagnosis of a coronary artery pseudoaneurysm following percutaneous transluminal coronary angioplasty. *Am. Heart J.*, **125**, 880–882.

68. Caccione, J.G., K. Reddy, F. Richards, H. Sheehan and J.M. Hodgson, 1991, Combined intravascular ultrasound/angioplasty balloon catheter: Initial use during PTCA. *Cathet. Cardiovasc. Diagn.*, **24**, 99–101.

69. Isner, J.M., K. Rosenfield, D.W. Losordo, L. Rose, Jr. R.E. Langevin, S. Razvi and B.D. Kosowsky, 1991, Combination balloon-ultrasound imaging catheter for percutaneous transluminal angioplasty: Validation of imaging, analysis of recoil, and identification of plaque fracture. *Circulation*, **84**, 739–754.

70. Wolfe, C.L., M.A. Klette, R.V. Trask, D.A. Rothbaum, R.J. Landin, M.W. Ball, Z.I. Hodes and T.J. Linnemeier, 1994, Assessment of the results of percutaneous transluminal coronary angioplasty using an integrated ultrasound imaging-angioplasty catheter. *Cathet. Cardiovasc. Diagn.*, **32**, 108–112.

71. Mudra, H., V. Klauss, R. Blasini, M. Kroetz, J. Rieber, E. Regar and K. Theisen, 1994, Ultrasound guidance of Palmaz-Schatz intracoronary stenting with a combined intravascular ultrasound balloon catheter. *Circulation*, **90**, 1252–1261.

72. Cavaye, D.M., R.A. White, R.D. Lerman, G.E. Kopchock, M.R. Tabbara, F. Cormier and W.J. French, 1992, Usefulness of intravascular ultrasound imaging for detecting experimentally induced aortic dissection in dogs and for determining the effectiveness of endoluminal stenting. *Am. J. Cardiol.*, **69**, 705–707.

73. Schryver, T.E., J.J. Popma, K.M. Kent, M.B. Leon and G.S. Mintz, 1992, Use of intracoronary ultrasound to identify the true coronary lumen in chronic coronary dissection treated with intracoronary stenting. *Am. J. Cardiol.*, **69**, 107–108.

74. Laskey, W.K., S.T. Brady, W.G. Kussmaul, A.R. Waxler, J. Krol, H.C. Herrmann, J.W. Hirshfeld and C. Sehgal, 1993, Intravascular ultrasonographic assessment of the results of coronary artery stenting. *Am. Heart J.*, **125**, 1576–1583.

75. Nakamura, S., A. Colombo, A. Gaglione, Y. Almagor, S.L. Goldberg, L. Maiello, L. Finci and J.M. Tobis, 1994, Intracoronary ultrasound observations during stent implantation. *Circulation*, **89**, 26–34.

76. Colombo, A., P. Hall, S. Nakamura, Y. Almagor, L. Maiello, G. Martini, A. Gaglione, S.L. Goldberg and J.M. Tobis, 1995, Intracoronary stenting without anticoagulation accomplished with intravascular ultrasound guidance. *Circulation*, **19**, 1676–1688.

77. Serruys, P.W. and C. Di Mario, 1995, Who was thrombogenic, the stent or the doctor? (editorial). *Circulation*, **19**, 1891–1893.

78. Tenaglia, A.N., K. Kisslo, S. Kelly, M.A. Hamm, R. Crowley and C.J. Davidson, 1993, Ultrasound guide wire-directed stent deployment. *Am. Heart J.*, **125**, 1213–1216.

79. De Lezo, J.S., M. Romero, A. Medina, M. Pan, D. Pavlovic, R. Vaamonde, E. Hernandez, F. Melian, F.L. Rubio, J. Marrero, J. Segura, M. Irurita and J.A. Cabrera, 1993, Intracoronary ultrasound assessment of directional coronary atherectomy: Immediate and follow-up findings. *J. Am. Coll. Cardiol.*, **21**, 298–307.

80. Popma, J.J., G.S. Mintz, L.F. Satler, A.D. Pichard, K.M. Kent, Y.C. Chuang, F. Matar, T.A. Bucher, A.J. Merritt and M.B. Leon, 1993, Clinical and angiographic outcome after directional coronary atherectomy: A qualitative and quantitative analysis using coronary arteriography and intravascular ultrasound. *Am. J. Cardiol.*, **72**, 55E–64E.

81. Gibbons, H.G. and V.J. Dzau, 1994, The emerging concept of vascular remodeling. *New Engl. J. Med.*, **330**, 1431–1438.

82. Yock, P.G., P.J. Fitzgerald, T.G. Yang, J. McKenzie, M. Belef, N. Starksen, N.W. White, D.T. Linker and J.B. Simpson, 1990, Initial trials of a combined ultrasound imaging/mechanical atherectomy catheter (abstract). *J. Am. Coll. Cardiol.*, **15**, 105A.

83. Suneja, R., R.N. Nair, K.G. Reddy, Q. Rasheed, H.M. Sheehan and J.M. Hodgson, 1993, Mechanisms of angiographically successful directional coronary atherectomy: Evaluation by intracoronary ultrasound and comparison with transluminal coronary angioplasty. *Am. Heart J.*, **126**, 507–514.

84. Li, W., C. von Birgelen, C. Di Mario, E. Boersma, E.J. Gussenhoven, N. van der Putten and N. Bom, 1994, Semi-automatic contour detection for volumetric quantification of intracoronary ultrasound. In *Proc. Comput. Cardiol.*, pp. 277–280, IEEE.

85. von Birgelen, C., C. Di Mario, W. Li, E. Camenzind, Y. Ozaki, P.J. de Feyter, N. Bom and J.R.T.C. Roelandt, 1994, Volumetric quantification in intracoronary ultrasound: Validation of a new automatic contour detection method with integrated user interaction (abstract). *Circulation*, **90**, I-550.

86. Cavaye, D.M., M.R. Tabbara, G.E. Kopchok, T.E. Laas and R.A. White, 1991, Three dimensional vascular ultrasound imaging. *The American Surgeon*, **57**, 751–755.

87. Rosenfield, K., J. Kaufman, A.M. Pieczek, R.E. Langevin, P.E. Palefski, S.A. Pazvi and J.M. Isner, 1992, Human coronary and peripheral arteries: On-line three-dimensional reconstruction from two-dimensional intravascular us scans. *Radiology*, **184**, 823–832.

88. Herrington, D.M., T. Johnson, P. Santago and W.E. Snyder, 1992, Semi-automated boundary detection for intravascular ultrasound. In *Computers in Cardiology 1992*, pp. 103–106, Los Alamitos, CA, IEEE.

89. Rosenfield, K., D.W. Losordo, K. Ramaswamy, A. Pieczek, M. Kearney, J. Hogan and B.D. Kosowsky, 1991, Quantitative analysis of luminal cross-sectional area from 3-dimensional reconstructions of 2-dimensional intravascular ultrasound: Validation of a novel technique (abstract). *Circulation*, **84**, II-542.

90. Wenguang, L., W.J. Gussenhoven, Y. Zhong, S.H.K. The, C. Di Mario, S. Madretsma, F.V. Egmond, P.D. Feyter, H. Pieterman, H.V. Urk, H. Rijsterborgh and N. Bom, 1991, Validation of quantitative analysis of intravascular ultrasound images. *Int. J. Cardiac Imag.*, **6**, 247–253.

91. Lee, R.T., H.M. Loree, G.C. Cheng, E.H. Liegerman, N. Jaramillo and F.J. Schoen, 1993, Computational structural analysis based on intravascular ultrasound imaging before *in vitro* angioplasty: Prediction of plaque fracture locations. *J. Am. Coll. Cardiol.*, **21**, 777–782.

92. Dhawale, P.J., D.L. Wilson and J. McB Hodgson, 1993, *In vivo* estimation of elastic properties of arteries with intracoronary ultrasound. In *Proceedings of the Annual International Conference of the IEEE Engineering in Medicine and Biology Society, Volume 15*, pp. 204–205, Piscataway, NJ, IEEE.

93. Nishimura, R.A., W.D. Edwards, C.A. Warnes, G.S. Reeder, D.R. Holmes, A.J. Tajik and P.G. Yock, 1990, Intravascular ultrasound imaging: *In vitro* validation and pathologic correlation. *J. Am. Coll. Cardiol.*, **16**, 145–154.

94. Rosenfield, K., D.W. Losordo, K. Ramaswamy, J.O. Pastore, R.E. Langevin, S. Razvi, B.D. Kosowsky and J.M. Isner, 1991, Three-dimensional reconstruction of human coronary and peripheral arteries from images recorded during two-dimensional intravascular ultrasound examination. *Circulation*, **84**, 1938–1956.

95. Pasterkamp, G., M.S. van der Heiden, M.J. Post, B. Ter Haar Romeny, W.P.T.M. Mali and C. Borst, 1993, Discrimination of the intravascular lumen and dissections in a single 30 MHz ultrasound image: Use of confounding blood backscatter to advantage. *Radiology*, **187**, 871–872.

96. Mottley, J.G., R.M. Glueck, J.E. Perez, B.E. Sobel and J.G. Miller, 1984, Regional differences in the cyclic variation of myocardial backscatter that parallel regional differences in contractile performance. *J. Acoust. Soc. Am.*, **76**, 1617–1623.

97. Rijsterborgh, H., F. Mastik, C.T. Lancee, P.D. Verdouw, J.R.C.T. Roelandt and N. Bom, 1993, Ultrasound myocardial integrated backscatter signal processing: Frequency domain versus time domain. *Ultrasound Med. Biol.*, **19**, 211–219.

98. Wickline, S.A., J.G. Miller, D. Rechia, A.M. Sharkey, L. Bridal and D. Christy, 1994, Beyond intravascular imaging: Quantitative ultrasonic tissue characterization of vascular pathology. In *IEEE Ultrasonics Symp.*, pp. 1589–1597, IEEE.

99. Insana, M.F., R.F. Wagner, B.S. Garra, D.G. Brown and T.H. Shawker, 1986, Analysis of ultrasound image texture via generalized Rician statistics. *Optical Engineering*, **25**, 743–748.

100. Momenan, R., R.F. Wagner, B.S. Garra, M.H. Loew and M.F. Insana, 1994, Image staining and differential diagnosis of ultrasound scans based on the Mahalanobis distance. *IEEE Trans. Med. Imaging*, **13**, 37–47.

101. Muzzolini, R., Y.H. Yang and R. Pierson, 1993, Multiresolution texture segmentation with application to diagnostic ultrasound images. *IEEE Trans. Med. Imaging*, **12**, 108–123.

102. Muzzolini, R., Y. Yee-Hong and R. Pierson, 1994, Texture characterization using robust statistics. *Pattern Recognition*, **27**, 119–134.

103. Durikovic, R., K. Kaneda and H. Yamashita, 1994, Texture approach to dynamic contour following. *Transactions of the Information Processing Society of Japan*, **35**, 1732–1738.

104. Dhawale, P.J., Q. Rasheed, N. Griffin, D.L. Wilson and J. McB Hodgson, 1993, Intracoronary ultrasound plaque volume quantification. In *Computers in Cardiology*, pp. 121–124, Los Alamitos, CA, IEEE.

105. Sonka, M., V. Hlavac and R. Boyle, 1993, *Image Processing, Analysis, and Machine Vision*. Chapman and Hall, London, New York.

106. White, C.J., S.R. Ramee, T.J. Collins, A. Jain and J.E. Mesa, 1992, Ambiguous coronary angiography: Clinical utility of intravascular ultrasound. *Cath. Cardiovasc. Diagn.*, **26**, 200–203.

107. Mudra, H., R. Blasini, V. Klauss, E. Regar, J. Rieber, A. Konig, M. Roth, R. von Essen and K. Theisen, 1992, Diameter measurements after balloon angioplasty by intravascular ultrasound and quantitative coronary angiography: Reasons for discrepancy (abstract). *Circulation*, **88**, I–411.

108. Kovach, J.A., G.S. Mintz, K.M. Kent, A.D. Pichard, L.F. Satler, J.J. Popma and M.B. Leon, 1993, Serial intravascular studies indicate that chronic recoil is an important mechanism of restenosis following transcatheter therapy (abstract). *J. Am. Coll. Cardiol.*, **21**, 484A.

109. Mintz, G.S., J.A. Kovach, A.D. Pichard, K.M. Kent, L.F. Satler, J.J. Popma, J.A. Painter, K. Forgan and M.B. Leon, 1994, Geometric remodeling is the predominant mechanism of clinical restenosis after coronary angioplasty (abstract). *J. Am. Coll. Cardiol.*, **23**, 138A.

110. Di Mario, C., R. Gil, E. Camenzind, Y. Ozaki, C. von Birgelen, V. Umans, P. de Jaegere, P.J. de Feyter, J.R.T.C. Roelandt and P.W. Serruys, 1995, Quantitative assessment with intracoronary ultrasound of the mechanisms of restenosis after percutaneous transluminal coronary angioplasty and directional coronary atherectomy. *Am. J. Cardiol.*, **75**, 772–777.

111. Roelandt, J.R.T.C., C. Di Mario, N.G. Pandian, W. Li, D. Keane, C.S. Slager, P.J. de Feyter and P.W. Serruys, 1994, Three-dimensional reconstruction of intracoronary ultrasound images: Rationale, approaches, problems and directions. *Circulation*, **90**, 1044–1055.

112. von Birgelen, C., C. Di Mario, W. Li, F. Prati, N. Bom, J.R.T.C. Roelandt and P.W. Serruys, 1995, Three-dimensional reconstruction of intracoronary ultrasound images: Technical approaches, clinical applications, and current limitations in the assessment of vessel dimensions. In A.M. Gotto Jr., C. Lenfant, A.L. Catapano and R. Paoletti, editors, *Multiple Risk Factors in Cardiovascular Disease: Vascular and Organ Protection*, pp. 267–287. Kluver, Dordrecht, Boston, London.

113. Rosenfield, K., J. Kaufman, D.W. Losordo and J.M. Isner, 1992, Lumen cast analysis: A quantitative format to expedite on-line analysis of 3D intravascular ultrasound images (abstract). *J. Am. Coll. Cardiol.*, **19**, 115A.

114. Rosenfield, K., J. Kaufman, A. Pieczek, R.E. Langevin, S. Razvi and J.M. Ilsner, 1992, Real-time three-dimensional reconstruction of intravascular ultrasound images of iliac arteries. *Am. J. Cardiol.*, **70**, 412–415.

115. Coy, K.M., J.C. Park, M.C. Fishbein, T. Laas, G.A. Diamond, L. Adler, G. Maurer and R.J. Siegel, 1992, *In vitro* validation of three-dimensional intravascular ultrasound for the evaluation of arterial injury after balloon angioplasty. *J. Am. Coll. Cardiol.*, **20**, 692–700.

116. Prati, F., C. Di Mario, C. von Birgelen, R. Gil, P.J. de Feyter, P.J. de Jaegere, W. van der Giessen and P.W. Serruys, 1995, Usefulness of on-line 3D reconstruction for stent implantation (abstract). *J. Am. Coll. Cardiol.*, **25**, 9A–10A.

117. Dhawale, P.J., D.L. Wilson and J.M. Hodgson, 1994, Optimal data acquisition for volumetric intracoronary ultrasound. *Cathet. Cardiovasc. Diagn.*, **32**, 288–299.

118. von Birgelen, C., C. Di Mario, W. Li, J.C.H. Schuurbiers, C.J. Slager, P. Ruygrok, F. Prati, P.J. De Feyter, P.W. Serruys and J.R.T.C. Roelandt, 1995, Clinical applications of a new computerized method measuring coronary artery dimensions by three-dimensional intracoronary ultrasound (abstract). *Eur. Heart J.*, **16** — Supplement.

119. Dhawale, P.J., Q. Rasheed, J. Berry and J.M. Hodgson, 1994, Quantification of lumen and plaque volume with ultrasound: Accuracy and short term variability in patients (abstract). *Circulation*, **90**, I–164.

120. Dhawale, P.J., Q. Rasheed, W. Mecca, R. Nair and J.M. Hodgson, 1993, Analysis of plaque volume during DCA using a volumetrically accurate three-dimensional ultrasound technique (abstract). *Circulation*, **88**, I–550.

121. Galli, F.C., K. Sudhir, A.K. Kao, P.J. Fitgerald and P.G. Yock, 1992, Direct measurement of plaque volume by three-dimensional ultrasound: Potential and pitfalls (abstract). *J. Am. Coll. Cardiol.*, **19**, 115A.

122. Smucker, M.L., D. Kil, W.S. Sarnat and P.F. Howard, 1992, Is three-dimensional reconstruction a gimmick or a useful clinical tool? Experience in coronary atherectomy (abstract). *J. Am. Coll. Cardiol.*, **19**, 115A.

123. Harrison, D.G., C.W. White, L.F. Hiratzka, D.B. Doty, D.H. Barnes, C.L. Eastham and M.L. Marcus, 1984, The value of lesion cross-sectional area determined by quantitative coronary angiography in assessing the physiologic significance of proximal left anterior descending coronary arterial stenoses. *Circulation*, **69**, 1111–1119.

124. von Birgelen, C., C. Di Mario, F. Prati, N. Bruining, W. Li, P.J. De Feyter and J.R.T.C. Roelandt, 1995, Intracoronary ultrasound: Three-dimensional reconstruction techniques. In C. Di Mario, P.J. De Feyter and J.R.T.C. Roelandt, editors, *Quantitative Coronary Imaging*, pp. 181–197. Barjesteh, Meeuwes & Co., Rotterdam.

125. Mintz, G.S., M.B. Keller and F.G. Fay, 1992, Motorized IVUS transducer pull-back permits accurate quantitative axial measurements (abstract). *Circulation*, **86**, I–323.

126. Di Mario, C., C. von Birgelen, F. Prati, B. Soni, W. Li, N. Bruining, P.J. de Jaegere, P.J. de Feyter, P.W. Serruys and J.R.T.C. Roelandt, 1995, Three-dimensional reconstruction of two-dimensional intracoronary ultrasound: Clinical or research tool? *Br. Heart J.*, **73** (Suppl. 2), 26–32.

127. Pandian, N.G., N.C. Nanda, S.L. Schwartz, P. Fan, Q.L. Cao, R. Sanyal, T.L. Hsu, B. Mumm, H. Wollschlager and A. Weintraub, 1992, Three-dimensional and four-dimensional transesophageal echocardiographic imaging of the heart and aorta in humans using computed tomographic imaging probe. *Echocardiography*, **9**, 677–687.

128. Roelandt, J.R.T.C., F.J. Ten Cate, W.B. Vletter and M.A. Taams, 1994, Ultrasonic dynamic three-dimensional visualization of the heart using a vario-plane transesophageal imaging transducer (Varioplane Echo-CT). *J. Am. Soc. Echocardiogr.*, **7**, 217–229.

129. Wollschlager, H., A.M. Zeiher, A. Geibel, W. Kasper and H. Just, 1992, Transesophageal echo-computer tomography: Computional reconstruction of any desired view of the beating heart. In *Cardiovascular Imaging by Ultrasound*, pp. 461–468, Dordrecht. Kluwer Academic Publishers.

130. Masotti, L. and R. Pini, 1993, Three-dimensional imaging. In *Advances in Ultrasound Techniques and Instrumentation*, pp. 69–77, New York. Churchill Livingstone.

131. Chandrasekaran, K., A.J. D'Adamo and C.M. Sehgal, 1992, Three-dimensional reconstruction of intravascular ultrasound images. In *Intravasc. Ultrasound Imag.*, pp. 141–147, New York, Churchill-Livingston.

132. Kitney, R., L. Moura and K. Straughan, 1989, 3D visualization of arterial structures using ultrasound and voxel modelling. *Int. J. Cardiac Imag.*, **4**, 135–143.

133. von Birgelen, C., C. Di Mario, N. van der Putten, W. Li, R. Gil, F. Prati, J. Ligthart, E. Camenzind, Y. Ozaki, P.W. Serruys and J.R.T.C. Roelandt, 1995, Quantification in three-dimensional intracoronary ultrasound: Importance of image acquisition and segmentation. *Cardiologie*, **2**, 67–72.

134. Hausmann, D., G. Friedrich, K. Sudhir, W.L. Mullen, B. Soni, P.J. Fitzgerald and P.G. Yock, 1994, 3D intravascular ultrasound imaging with automated border detection using 2.9 F catheters (abstract). *J. Am. Coll. Cardiol.*, **23**, 174A.

135. Prati, F., C. Di Mario, C. von Birgelen, R. Gil, J. Ligthart, P. Ruygrok, J.R.T.C. Roelandt, P.J. de Feyter and P.W. Serruys, 1995, On-line automated lumen volumen measurement with 3D intracoronary ultrasound during coronary interventions (abstract). *J. Am. Coll. Cardiol.*, **25**, 345A.

136. Sonka, M., X. Zhang, M. Siebes, S. DeJong, C.R. McKay and S.M. Collins, 1995, Automated segmentation of coronary wall and plaque from intravascular ultrasound image sequences. In *Computers in Cardiology 1994*, pp. 281–284, Los Alamitos, CA, IEEE.

137. Sonka, M., W. Liang, X. Zhang, S. DeJong, S.M. Collins and C.R. McKay, 1995, Three-dimensional automated segmentation of coronary wall and plaque from intravascular ultrasound pullback sequences. In *Computers in Cardiology 1995*, Los Alamitos, CA, IEEE. In press.

138. Li, W., E.J. Gussenhoven, Y. Zhong, S.H.K. The, C. Di Mario, S. Madretsma, F. van Egmond, P.J. de Feyter, H. Pieterman, H. van Urk, H. Rijsterborgh and N. Bom, 1991, Validation of quantitative analysis of intravascular ultrasound images. *Int. J. Cardiac Imag.*, **6**, 247–254.

139. Li, W., J.G. Bosch, Y. Zhong, H. van Urk, E.J. Gussenhoven, F. Mastik, F. van Egmond, H. Rijstenborgh, J.H.C. Reiber and N. Bom, 1993, Image segmentation and 3D reconstruction of intravascular ultrasound images. *Acoustic Imaging*, **20**, 489–496.

140. Sonka, M., X. Zhang, M. Siebes, M.S. Bissing, S. DeJong, S.M. Collins and C.R. McKay, 1994, Semi-automated detection of coronary arterial wall and plaque borders in intravascular ultrasound images (abstract). *Circulation*, **90**, I-550.

141. Sonka, M., X. Zhang, M. Siebes, M.S. Bissing, S. DeJong, S.M. Collins and C.R. McKay, 1996, Segmentation of intravascular ultrasound images: A knowledge-based approach. *IEEE Trans. Med. Imaging*, **15**, in press.

142. Li, S., W.N. McDicken and P.R. Hoskins, 1993, Blood vessel diameter measurement by ultrasound. *Physiol. Meas.*, **14**, 291–297.
143. Di Mario, C., S. Madretsma, D. Linker, S.H.K. The, N. Bom, P.W. Serruys, E.J. Gussenhoven and J.R.T.C. Roelandt, 1993, The angle of incidence of the ultrasonic beam: A critical factor for the image quality in intravascular ultrasound. *Am. Heart J.*, **125**, 442–448.
144. Slager, C.J., M. Laban, C. von Birgelen, R. Krams, J.A.F. Oomen, A. den Boer, W. Li, P.J. de Feyter, P.W. Serruys and J.R.T.C. Roelandt, 1995, ANGUS: A new approach to three-dimensional reconstruction of geometry and orientation of coronary lumen and plaque by combined use of coronary angiography and ivus (abstract). *J. Am. Coll. Cardiol.*, **25**, 144A.
145. Waligora, M.J., M.J. Vonesh, S.P. Wiet and D.D. McPherson, 1994, Effect of vascular curvature on three-dimensional reconstruction of intravascular ultrasound images (abstract). *Circulation*, **90**, I–277.

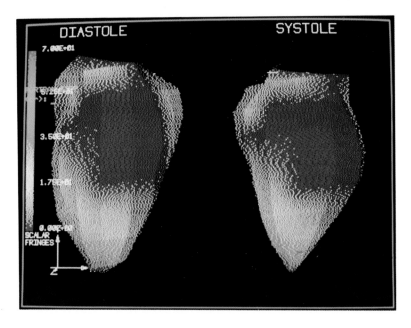

COLOR PLATE I. *See* H. Azhari, R. Beyar and S. Sideman, Figure 9, page 19.

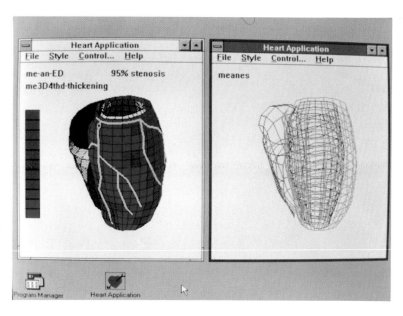

COLOR PLATE II. *See* H. Azhari, R. Beyar and S. Sideman, Figure 10, page 19.